TO LIVE IS TO WORSHIP
BIOETHICS AND THE BODY OF CHRIST

The 2006
J. J. Thiessen
Lectures

TO LIVE IS TO WORSHIP
BIOETHICS AND THE BODY OF CHRIST

Joel James Shuman

CMU Press
Winnipeg, Manitoba
2007

CMU Press
500 Shaftesbury Blvd.
Winnipeg, Manitoba R3P 2N2

CMU Press is an academic publisher of scholarly, reference, and general interest books at Canadian Mennonite University. Books from CMU Press address and inform interests and issues vital to the university, its constituency, and society. Areas of specialization include Mennonite studies, and works that are church-oriented or theologically engaged. For more information about CMU Press contact cmupress@cmu.ca or tel. 204.487.3300 or visit www.cmu.ca/publications.

Some of the material in Chapter 2 appeared in a different form in *Reclaiming the Body: Christians and the Faithful Use of Modern Medicine* (2006), by Joel James Shuman and Brian Volck, and is used with the permission of Brazos Press.

Cover design: Diana Crosby

Library and Archives Canada Cataloguing in Publication

Shuman, Joel James
To live is to worship : bioethics and the body of Christ / Joel James Shuman.

(The 2006 J.J. Thiessen lectures)
Includes bibliographical references.
ISBN 978-0-920718-79-7

1. Medicine--Religious aspects--Christianity. 2. Body, Human--Religious aspects--Christianity. 3. Worship. I. Title. II. Series: J.J. Thiessen lectures 2006

BT732.S483 2007 261.5'61 C2007-903095-5

Printed in Canada by
Christian Press
Winnipeg, Manitoba

CONTENTS

The 2006 J. J. Thiessen Lectures
were presented at
Canadian Mennonite University
on October 17-18, 2006

FOREWORD

The American philosopher Stanley Cavell suggests that the dominant image of the body in contemporary western social orders such as ours is that of a limitation that leaves us feeling "chafed by our own skin." I think this striking image instructively helps to situate Joel Shuman's attempt to develop a theologically robust discussion of medicine and bioethics. Like Cavell, Shuman argues that much of our thought is distorted by an inadequate conception of the body as something that chafes against us. In particular, he suggests that our understanding of both medicine and worship typically assumes that the body is essentially a liability or limitation that is ideally overcome.

I suspect most of us are not accustomed to thinking of medicine and worship as having much, if anything, to do with each other. To the extent that we do, we tend to think of worship as a therapeutic aid that enables us to negotiate the crises of our lives so forcefully captured by certain medical conditions. But such a conception of worship is limited just to the extent that it neglects the sense in which Christian worship is a formation of the body. It is this sense of worship that Joel Shuman develops in these 2006 J.J. Thiessen Lectures. And we will see that it has profound implications for how we understand the ends of the body associated with medicine and health.

According to Shuman, medicine and worship are best understood in terms of what has been called "crafts of place." They name a set of interdependent and concretely located practices that serve to inform and make intelligible the lives and deaths of essentially embodied and interdependent creatures. In particular, Shuman argues that medicine and worship are to be situated in that complex place called church. It is important to note, however, that he is not merely suggesting that medicine be located in the context of worship, as if what is meant by worship is relatively straightforward. Rather, Shuman's discussion equally involves a reflection on the lamentable fact that worship all too often takes place as if its location in the church is insignificant, or at most optional. Indeed, the heart of his argument turns upon the suggestion that such a deficient conception of worship is inextricably bound up with some of our characteristic difficulties in negotiating the world of modern medicine. According to Shuman, worship is not a vehicle for expressing our deepest held feelings, but a radically transformative process whereby we are taken up into and redefined by participation in the very body of Christ. In particular, worship names the work of the church through which we learn to be appropriately dependent upon one another and on God in particular. And such a vision of worship cannot help but inform a radically different approach to bioethics than the rather legalistic and bureaucratic field it has largely become.

If you have come to this book on medical ethics looking for formulas designed to calculate solutions to difficult ethical questions and so-called moral dilemmas, let me apologize in advance, because I'm afraid you have come to the wrong place. But if you are willing to entertain a fascinating and wide-ranging set of theological and cultural reflections on how the body is formed through practices of worship and medicine, then I'm confident that you will not be disappointed.

Chris K. Huebner
Canadian Mennonite University
April 2007

One

What We Cannot *Not* Do: Why Worship *Is* Bioethics—and Vice Versa

Now is the time to endure; then will be the day of consolation . . . . We say, indeed, that we desire the kingdom of heaven, yet we are not solicitous for the means whereby it is attained.—Saint Basil the Great[1]

The grace that is the health of creatures can only be held in common.
In healing the scattered members come together.
In health the flesh is graced, the holy enters the world.—Wendell Berry[2]

I begin by juxtaposing these very different sayings, because that juxtaposition expresses nicely the real tension faithful Christians have felt and should continue to feel when they begin talking about things like health and medicine and worship and bioethics. The tension of which I speak is one concrete manifestation of what theologians and theologically interested New Testament scholars in particular refer to as the dialectical tension between the eschatological "now and the not yet." This is a tension between on the one hand finding the kingdom of God already present in the world as it now is or could be, and on the other hand having to remain content only to anticipate the kingdom as we believe it will be in the age to come.

The former saying, by the fourth-century theologian and bishop, Saint Basil the Great, suggests the possibility that this life is of little ultimate importance and that our focus should be on preparing ourselves for the life to come, for there and there only is our true flourishing to be found. The task of this life is to participate with God in the reordering of our desires, so that our meeting with God in the life to come will be a happy one. The latter saying, by the contemporary poet, essayist, and farmer Wendell Berry, suggests that the blessings of God are present in considerable measure to this life and that we would do well to respond to and cultivate that presence—also by reordering our desires. By God's grace, Berry implies, a significant measure of flourishing is available to us now through such cultivation. In these lectures I will argue that both sayings are correct, and that it is proper and fitting for Christians to use medicine and the other applied sciences to pursue and enjoy a significant measure of happiness and health in this life, while at the same time recognizing that happiness and health can be enjoyed in their fullness only in the age to come, when the reign of God is consummated.

For the theologically attentive listener, the assertion that both sayings are correct rightfully raises several questions. What does it mean for Christians to be a people who proclaim thankfully the goodness of the gifts of human life and health as integral to our enjoyment of an abundant creation, while at the same time professing to worship a crucified God whose self-emptying example we are called to imitate? How may we account for the fact that we are at once a people who have always been concerned to care for the sick because we worship a Lord who was known especially for his ministry of healing and his solidarity with the afflicted, while at the same time acknowledging that because of our self-inflicted alienation from God, sickness and death ultimately will have their way this side of the consummation of history? How far may we go in our struggle against suffering, sickness, and death? How, in short, does our worship of the triune God comport with the possibilities afforded by modern medicine and the other applied biological sciences? These are the questions I hope, indirectly if not directly, to address.

The moment we begin thinking about proper or improper uses of modern medicine we find ourselves on terrain typically inhabited by bioethicists. And so we must begin by expressing a strong reservation. Any theologically helpful conversation about these matters—that is, about worship and bioethics—needs to begin by explicitly resisting the temptation to move forward from this point assuming that "worship" and "bioethics" name discrete discourses that need now to be brought into conversation, preferably through consultation with experts in the respective fields. To be sure, such disciplines and such experts do exist, and both make valuable contributions to conversations such as the one we are engaged in. Yet, to begin and end with those contributions would be unnecessarily to reify these categories (that is, "worship" and "bioethics") and attenuate our discussion in unhappy ways. For as the title of this first lecture indicates, I wish to argue that there is a sense in which worship *is* bioethics, and vice versa.

We are creatures. And although we are created in the image of the triune God and invited and enabled by God's grace to enter eternity and participate in the mutual love among Father, Son, and Holy Spirit, we do so as living bodies. In this life and the next, we are never properly less than our bodies. Always and everywhere, we exist as fragments of animated earth, entwined in complex webs of contingent interdependent relationships with particular people, places, and things. These relationships are constitutive of our very being. They shape and circumscribe our identities. And because we and the creation of which we are a part are so shaped and circumscribed, and because we bear the marks of our self-inflicted alienation from our Creator and Sustainer, we are required to labour for our survival and to endure all kinds of conflict, including conflict with sickness and death, until we return to the dust from which we came. That is our fate.[3]

We are creatures. But we are also, at least in the broadest sense, worshippers. Whether we are conscious of it or not, we live our lives always oriented toward some Good or goods. Because we possess intellect and will as well as appetite, we have the capacity to make judgements about these goods. Just so, we are accountable for these things.[4] That it does not usually occur to us to affix to the orientation of our affections the same name we give to what Christians do when they gather on the Lord's Day is of little consequence. Nicholas Lash says:

> It is taken for granted, in sophisticated circles, that no one worships God these days except the reactionary and the simple-minded. This innocent self-satisfaction tells us little more, however, than that those exhibiting it do not name as "God" the gods they worship. In fact, whatever names we give to things, we worship things (especially ourselves) as naturally and as spontaneously as we breathe and speak. We have no option but to have our hearts set somewhere, to hold something sacred.[5]

In making this claim, I do not believe Lash is taking unwarranted liberty in his description of worship. Later in the same essay, he says that "the word 'god' is not a proper noun. It is the common name for whatever people worship, whatever they take to be divine. And 'being divine' is not like being fat or thin, being British or short-sighted. It is more like being heard or seen. Something is heard or seen if someone hears or sees it. Something is divine if someone worships it."[6] The philosopher who said that "Everything is full of gods" was in this sense correct; our gods are pretty much where we find them. There is abundant precedent, even within Christian tradition, for this way of thinking: to take but one example, Martin Luther said almost five hundred years ago that "A god means that from which we are to expect all good and to which we are to take refuge in all distress, so that to have a God is nothing else than to trust and believe. . . . That now, I say, upon which you set your heart and put your trust is properly your god."[7]

The question then is not one of whether we worship, but of whom or what we worship, and how. For while worship may well come naturally to us, the faithful worship of the God of Israel, Jesus, and the church does not. No one, says Luther, "has ever been so reprobate as not to institute and observe some divine worship; every one has set up as his special god whatever he looked to for blessings, help, and comfort."[8] The "special gods" of today are seldom made of wood, stone, or metal, but are no less real than their ancient counterparts. As Lash reminds us:

> All human beings have their hearts set somewhere, hold something sacred, worship at some shrine. We are spontaneously idolatrous—where by "idolatry," I mean the worship of some creature, the setting of the heart on some particular thing (usually oneself). For most of us, there is no single creature that is the object of our faith. Our hearts are torn, dispersed, distracted. We are (to use the seventeenth-century term) polytheists. And none of us is so self-transparent as to know quite where, in fact, our hearts are set.[9]

The Good or goods toward which we orient ourselves; the relationships into which we are born and the associations we form; the paths we take; the appetites we strive to satisfy; and the loves we pursue all make our lives as bodies what they are. And because we are forever making or failing to make judgements about these matters, judgements for which we are accountable, we are always "doing" bioethics, for that, ultimately, is what bioethics is: the discipline of making practical judgements about the body and its goods. Per chance or per force, these judgements cannot be other than a matter of worship, which is but a different way to say that worship and bioethics are both aspects of the same reality. As Wendell Berry puts it, "The question of human limits, of the proper definition and place of human beings within the order of creation, finally rests upon our attitude toward our biological existence, the life of the body in this world."[10] The things we believe constitute a life that is properly human, and the way we judge certain kinds of actions as properly human or not are functions of what we believe about what it means to be human and how we should occupy our place in the larger scheme of things. Thus nothing less is at stake (in understanding how properly to live as bodies in relationship to the earth and to other bodies) than our health and salvation: "by understanding accurately his proper place in creation, a man may be made whole."[11]

Regardless of whom or what we worship, then, our quest for health and the questions attending that quest are irreducibly theological. As Berry reminds us, the English words healthy, whole, and holy have a common linguistic ancestry.[12] We cannot attend properly to the questions of how to pursue, restore, or maintain our health—by any means—without attending as well to how those means comport or not with what we believe about our place in the creation and about the attendant obligations we have to each other and to the rest of creation.[13] For those of us who profess to be Christians and say we believe the very being of the universe to be constituted by the mutual love shared among the persons of the triune God, this suggests that the quest for health can never be reduced to a consideration of the proper uses of medicine in service to the desires of an isolated, autonomous individual; for the very idea of a healthy isolated, autonomous individual—an individual whose desires are simply his or her own—is fundamentally nonsensical.[14]

Saint Paul reminds his readers in Corinth of this when (in considering a somewhat different practical matter) he tells them "your body is a temple of the Holy Spirit within you, which you have from God, and . . . you are not your own. For you were bought with a price; therefore glorify God in your body" (1 Corinthians 6:19-20). The Corinthians, you will remember, were a people divided along lines of class, wealth, and education; and there were those in their community who believed that their knowledge of Christ freed them from Judaism's conventional moral obligations. Paul is quick to dispel this belief, reminding them that their bodies have been claimed by God and united to God and each other. Similarly, any questions we as Christians ask about how properly to use medicine or any other biotechnology must account for the claims God makes upon us in making our bodies part of the one body of Christ. In doing so, we enter into a conversation long since begun and from which we have much to learn. Saint Basil the Great, writing the "Long Rules" for his ascetical community—the saying with which I began is from the Preface to that treatise—concludes those rules with a consideration of a broad version of the question these lectures presuppose: "whether recourse to the medical art is in keeping with the practice of piety."[15] He offers a lengthy, and from our perspective, surprisingly relevant answer, which we do well to consider.

Basil seems concerned to counter explicitly two errors which were no doubt common in his day, and which are at least analogous to mistakes that stand in the way of a faithful Christian use of modern medicine and the other applied sciences today. Given the contemporary North Atlantic obsession with all things medical, the first of these errors seems initially much less relevant to the contemporary situation. I speak here of the *in principle* rejection of the art of medicine, on grounds that its use displays a weakness of faith or the absence of piety. Basil denies this is the case, and offers a compelling argument that turns out to be an effective antidote, not simply to the mistake of rejecting medicine as irreligious, but also to the mistaken Gnostic tendencies of contemporary North Atlantic culture to segregate the spiritual from the material (or physical) and behave as if the two realms are, if related at all, only tangentially so. Basil shows us that this is tantamount to a denial of the goodness of creation.

Basil counts medicine among the arts, various kinds of disciplined human work done to complement and perfect the essential goodness of creation and to redress the effects of its brokenness. The arts, he says, are "God's gift to us, remedying the deficiencies of [presumably fallen] nature" (330). Medicine "has been vouchsafed us by God, who directs our whole life as a cure for the soul, to guide us in the removal of what is superfluous and in the addition of what is lacking" (331). His primary metaphor for medicine is agriculture. After the fall, the superabundance of creation was compromised, and it became necessary for women and men to work with the earth to encourage it to produce a sufficiency of food. Our capacity to learn and to understand the workings of the creation, themselves God's gifts, made this possible. Similarly, medicine is a gift from God in response to another of the effects of our alienation from God. Sickness and death, Basil asserts, are among the marks of that alienation; if we had not fallen, we would have no need of medicine. Just so, he says, "when we were commanded to return to the earth whence we had been taken and were united to the pain-ridden flesh doomed to destruction because of sin and, for the same reason, also subject to disease, the medical art was given to us to relieve the sick, in some degree at least" (331).

That medicine can be and frequently is misused is of little consequence to Basil. To reject it on such grounds would be akin to refusing to eat because some food is grown by people of questionable motives, or under questionable conditions, or by way of practices that threaten the long term integrity of the earth. Some of us know for a fact that each of these concerns applies to at least some of our food, and we are rightly disturbed by this knowledge. However, the proper response is not to stop eating, but to do as much as we can to eat faithfully—to learn and understand the social history of the food available to us and, to the extent possible, to eat food grown in ways that do not damage the earth or the bodies of the women and men who work to grow it.

The abject silliness of the idea that we might refuse to eat because eating is inherently unfaithful or because some eat unfaithfully prompts us to consider another possibility, less extreme but no less problematic, which is that we proceed with our lives never thinking about such matters as eating or medicine because they are hopelessly corrupted "secular" concerns which are of no real consequence theologically. Just as Paul encountered the former attitude among the members of the "strong" party in Corinth, who justified their indifference to the fact that some of their meat had been sacrificed to idols by insisting that "food is for the stomach and the stomach for food" (1 Corinthians 6:13), modern Christians must face and resist the temptation to regard science and technology and the bodies they serve as purely instrumental, as if they have no moral or theological significance of their own. Many adherents to this position apparently think that the relationship of theology to medicine should be primarily a matter of studying the clinical efficacy of prayer, which is thereby turned into one therapeutic modality among others. This tendency, which is at once Gnostic and reductionist in a way that would make Ludwig Feuerbach proud, runs just beneath the surface of many contemporary accounts of the relationship between spirituality and medicine.[16]

Such thinking is wrongheaded precisely because it treats the body as belonging to a realm of secondary importance with which God is largely unconcerned. But Christian tradition reminds us that our bodies are real; so real, in fact, as to mediate our every relationship, including and perhaps especially our relationship to God. Because our bodies are real, the sickness and suffering we experience as part of this life are real. And because sickness and suffering are real, the performance of sickness and suffering and the care of the sick and suffering are fundamental ways of participating in the sacredness of God, for there is nothing in creation that exists outside the purview of God's grace. "Holistic" or "spiritual" care, then, is never less than bodies being present to and caring for other bodies, for God has *made us* bodies.

The assertion that we are to care for one another's bodies raises questions of how and how much; that is, the means by which and the extent to which we are to do so. And this brings us to a consideration of the second error Basil counters in his response, an unwarranted regard for the capacities of medicine. He says: "Whatever requires an undue amount of thought or trouble or involves a large expenditure of effort and causes our whole life to revolve, as it were, around solicitude for the flesh must be avoided by Christians."[17] If this was a legitimate concern for Christians in Basil's time, it is surely more so in our own. Modern medicine is so capable, and its cultural power so great, that it is altogether possible that our uses of medicine can corrupt our worship of God. We can readily make medicine part of our idolatry, either by worshipping the power of medicine or by making medicine complicit in our worship of ourselves.

Basil's explication of this possibility suggests that the proximate cause of such idolatry is an inappropriate—perhaps it would be better to say an excessive—desire to live comfortably. This desire is in some measure natural; none of us, after all, wants to suffer. Yet the failure to check its pursuit stems ultimately from the suspicion that suffering and death are the worst things that can happen to us, and that freedom from suffering in this life, to quote Jack Nicholson's character from the movie of the same name, is "as good as it gets."

Again we may gain some clarity from consulting Paul's Corinthian correspondence. In the discourse on the resurrection, with which he concludes the letter we call 1 Corinthians, the Apostle claims that the only thing that renders the cruciform way of Christian discipleship intelligible is the bodily resurrection of Jesus from the dead, by which God has secured our resurrection from the dead and the restoration of all creation. "If for this life only we have hoped in Christ," Paul explains, "we are of all people most to be pitied" (1 Corinthians 15:19). The acceptance of suffering of any kind, including that which afflicts us because of sickness, makes sense only in light of the resurrection of Jesus and the attendant commencement of the New Creation. For, as Paul says, "If the dead are not raised, 'let us eat and drink, for tomorrow we die'" (1 Corinthians 15:32).

This of course leaves us with a problem. If we presume with Basil both that the power of medicine to relieve suffering is a good and that it is possible to misuse or overuse that power, how do we go about determining what uses constitute such errors? Basil's answer is understandably incomplete and (to my mind) finally unsatisfying. Yet it points us in a useful direction. You will remember that earlier in his argument, Basil asserted that the goodness of medicine is an extension of its being a legitimate participant in the goodness of God's creation, which we are called to receive as a gift. One way of describing idolatry is that it is the treatment of creation or some aspect of creation as *sui generis* and good in and of itself, rather than as good by virtue of its participation in God. A faithful use of any aspect of creation always entails, in other words, an acknowledgement that the creation is God's gift and that we are not its owners but its caretakers. This acknowledgement, moreover, must always include more than mental or verbal assent; it must also be evidenced as intrinsic to the particular use of creation in question.

Medicine, says Basil, must therefore never be regarded as "wholly accountable for our state of health, but as redounding to the glory of God and as a parallel to the care of the soul" (332). The worst use one can make of medicine is to treat the art or its practitioners as the final cause of well-being, or to use it in the service of life shaped determinatively by the denial of our creatureliness and all that status entails. To do so is "the act of an irrational animal. This, nevertheless, is what we observe in the case of certain unhappy persons who do not hesitate to call their doctors their saviors" (333). The practice of medicine properly understood is at most a secondary participation in the saving work of God. Here Basil finds an analogy in the Old Testament story of the healing of King Hezekiah. Hezekiah, you may remember, was king of Judah when Assyria was completing the destruction of Israel and threatening to do the same to Judah. The author of 2 Kings tells us that in the midst of these developments Hezekiah contracted a serious illness that threatened his life.

Initially, Hezekiah was told by the prophet Isaiah that the illness afflicting him was fatal. In response to Isaiah's prophecy, Hezekiah prayed to God and was subsequently healed when his attendants applied a lump of figs to the affected area of his body (2 Kings 20:1-11). Basil's use of this story to make his point is fairly straightforward. The figs were a proximate cause, but neither sufficient nor final, for Hezekiah's healing. Rather, as the text makes clear, he was healed by God, who responded to the king's prayer by once again sending to him the prophet Isaiah, who directed the application of the figs. Even more interesting is the biblical text's suggestion that this healing transpired not simply as a reward for Hezekiah's faithfulness or even as an expression of God's love, but also as a manifestation of God's covenant loyalty to God's people, and specifically to the throne of David. Hezekiah, the text asserts, would play an instrumental role in repelling an impending attack on the city by the King of Assyria, thereby delaying the destruction of the city and affording the people yet another opportunity to repent.

Questions about the fittingness of Basil's reading of this particular story notwithstanding, his imaginative use of the biblical narrative to address what is for him and for us a contemporary question suggests some interesting possibilities. In his reading of the story of Hezekiah's healing, Basil gives a narrative display of his previously made general claims about the appropriate relationship of divine and human action as displayed in healings effected, or apparently effected, by the art of medicine. This turn to the biblical narrative suggests a way of anticipating and possibly refuting the claim or assumption that some (mis)use of technology or another is proper simply because it exists and has capriciously been named a gift from God by some person or group of persons who desire one or more of its effects. Rather, the first and most basic question to be asked of any given technology must be whether the story of its development and its proposed use(s) can readily be taken up into and made part of the broader narrative of the Christian God's saving work in history.

The general tendency of most contemporary North Atlantic Christians is precisely the opposite; that is, we unproblematically subsume the biblical narrative under the authority of our own stories and the pervasive cultural narratives that dominate our lives as moderns, thereby relegating God to a tightly circumscribed portion of our lives called "religion" or "spirituality."[18] This has come about as we have been shaped over time to treat two characteristically modern stories as canonical; that is, as being stories against which all others are to be measured. The first of these is the rise of the liberal democratic nation-state and the concomitant emergence of the liberal notion of the autonomous self. Unencumbered by dependence upon or attachment to the authority of tradition, the modern self is supposedly free to choose her own projects and pursue her own desires as she sees fit. The second is the story of what Gerald McKenny calls the "Baconian Project," the way of thinking, speaking, and living that emerges in the wake of the triumphs of modern science. This is the hyper-optimistic story of the capacities of technology to satisfy human wants and increase human freedom by freeing women and men from the bonds of contingency, particularly those contingencies that exist because of the body and its afflictions.[19] Taken together (McKenny essentially regards them as parts of the same story) these stories have the effect of rendering untenable any normative account of what it means to be human and live a human life, other than having the capacity to create and use technology in the service of untutored desire.

This tendency toward reversal—Hans Frei calls the subsumption of the biblical story under the authority of competing narratives the "Great Reversal"—is in part a matter of attention. The relative authority of the biblical and modern narratives is a function of the extent to which they take hold of our imaginations, which is in turn a function of the ways and extent to which we attend to them. Such attention includes but also exceeds our intentionality, for the narratives of modernity—the stories of unlimited freedom, prosperity, and progress—are the very cultural air we breathe. Michel de Certeau explains:

> Seized from the moment of awakening by the radio (the voice is the law), the listener walks all day through a forest of narrativities, journalistic, advertising and televised, which, at night, slip a few final messages under the door of sleep. More than the God recounted to us by the theologians of the past, these tales have a function of providence and predestination: they organize our work, our celebrations—even our dreams—in advance. Social life multiplies the gestures and modes of behaviours *imprinted* by the narrative models: it continually reproduces and stores up the "copies" of narratives.[20]

Only as our attention is redirected to the biblical narrative may we properly orient our lives; only as our lives are properly oriented can we properly love creation and the arts that make use of creation for our benefit. To love and use creation properly we must see it not simply as coming from God, but also as belonging to God and destined ultimately to return to and be consummated in God. For a partial sense of the difference this might make, I direct your attention to the life and work of the great American writer Flannery O'Connor, a devout Catholic Christian who spent a significant part of her short life dealing with a debilitating and ultimately fatal illness. In a letter to a friend, O'Connor wrote:

> To see Christ as God and man is probably no more difficult today than it has always been, even if today there seem to be more reasons to doubt. For you it may be a matter of not being able to accept what you call a suspension of the laws of the flesh and the physical, but for my part I think that when I know what the laws of the flesh and the physical really are, then I will know what God is. We know them as we see them, not as God sees them. For me it is the virgin birth, the Incarnation, the resurrection which are the true laws of the flesh and the physical. Death, decay, and destruction are the suspension of these laws. . . . The resurrection of Christ seems the high point in the law of nature.[21]

O'Connor was able to see creation through the lens of the resurrection of Jesus because her attention was properly directed and her affections properly formed by her immersion in the practices of Christian worship, through which she learned to re-enact and embody the story of God's surprising work in the world. Perhaps the most stunning vision of that work in O'Connor's fiction is found in the conclusion of her short story "Revelation," where the self-assured, comfortably middle class, and deeply prejudiced protagonist, Mrs. Turpin, is given a brief glimpse of God's subversive reign. As she stands beside the hog parlour on her farm, having just demanded that God justify an earlier incident that had called into question her comfortable view of the world, she sees something in the evening sky.

> She raised her hands from the side of the pen in a gesture hieratic and profound. A visionary light

> settled in her eyes. She saw the streak as a vast swinging bridge extending upward from the earth through a field of living fire. Upon it a vast hoard of souls were rumbling upward toward heaven. There were whole companies of white trash, clean for the first time in their lives, and bands of black[s] . . . in white robes, and battalions of freaks and lunatics shouting and clapping and leaping like frogs. And bringing up the end of the procession was a tribe of people whom she recognized at once as those who, like herself and Claud, had always had a little of everything and the God-given wit to use it right. She leaned forward to observe them closer. They were marching behind the others with great dignity, accountable as they had always been for good order and common sense and respectable behavior. They alone were on key. Yet she could see by their shocked and altered faces that even their virtues were being burned away.[22]

Creation and the arts that extend from creation are God's gifts to us, but they cannot and will not save us in any ultimate sense. Only God saves. Life can be lived in gratitude and treated as a gift, even in the face of less than happy circumstances, because of the promise that the God who raised Jesus from death to life rules history and has given us a glimpse into its consummation. The seer of another Revelation offers us a picture of history's consummation, saying: "See, the home of God is among mortals./ He will dwell with them as their God;/ they will be his peoples,/ and God himself will be with them;/ he will wipe every tear from their eyes./ Death will be no more;/ mourning and crying and pain will be no more,/ for the first things have passed away."[23] This is health in its fullness: God dwelling with women and men in a renewed creation, free from animus, free from violence, free from suffering, free from death. It is the anticipation of that reality that enables us fully to live in this one, to be bodily present in loving service one to another, a presence that encompasses both worship and bioethics. And until history is brought to its glorious consummation, for what greater flourishing can we hope?

Two

Archai, Exousiai, Iatroi?: Naming Medicine among the Principalities and Powers[24]

In the first lecture I entered into conversation with Saint Basil, who suggested in his "Long Rules" that, although the art of medicine was a real good, it was at the same time susceptible to being misused or overused in ways that were tantamount to idolatry. Such misuses, he claimed, stem from an undue "solicitude for the flesh" which has its origin in our natural, and for the most part healthy, desire to avoid pain and suffering. Yet, to allow this desire free rein is to render ourselves potentially dependent upon this art and its human practitioners in a way that mitigates the proper ordering of affections acquired through the worship of the Christian God. In this lecture I want to argue that this mitigation is in large part a matter of power.

Power is simply the capacity of a subject to have an effect on an object.[25] Some philosophers go so far as to claim that power is an irreducible aspect of all human relationships, a point I am unprepared to challenge here.[26] In every human interaction, the question of the imposition of one party's will upon another is forever potential, if not already present. This is no less true in modern, liberal cultures like our own than in those societies we call totalitarian. This is not to deny the fairly obvious difference between liberalism and totalitarianism so much as it is to call attention to the ubiquity in all human relations of questions about the role and limits of power.[27] In liberal cultures like those in contemporary North America, power legitimates itself not so much by coercion as by co-option, by persuading those others it seeks to discipline that the wielders of power are the benevolent stewards of knowledge and skill to be exercised for the good of the disciplined.[28] There is thus an ineluctable relationship of power and knowledge. In other words, we confer authority upon people and institutions we regard as powerful mainly because we believe they know things we do not about the way the world is or could be—things that will make our lives better by granting us access to the things we want.[29] This seems to me one way of describing the constellation of practices we call modern medicine.

Volumes have been written about the power medicine wields in modern societies.[30] We cede a tremendous amount of authority to physicians and other representatives of the medical industry, not simply because we are afraid of illness or do not like to be ill, but also because we are convinced these men and women know things about our bodies that are, in the potential or actual presence of illness, essential to our well-being. We believe, in other words, that they hold in their hands, drugs, and machines the very power of life and death. This high regard, moreover, is normally not misplaced, for these women and men do seemingly magical things for us, preserving our lives and helping us function better than we would or could without their help.

At the same time, however, we tend to be ambivalent about granting so much power to medicine and its representatives. Our ambivalence comes not so much from our distrust of these particular men and women, but because the act of entrusting our lives to them makes us acutely aware of our extensive, persistent vulnerability. In our weakest and neediest moments, we discover a troubling dependence upon a group of relative strangers whose presence to our lives is mediated by a complex and frequently faceless bureaucracy. Just to the extent we have come to see ourselves as autonomous individuals who possess the capacity to exert certain kinds of power, our dependence calls into question our very being.

It is important to repeat that our discomfort with the power of medicine does not consist primarily as a suspicion of the motives of the women and men who are the face of the profession. To be sure, there are plenty of physicians, nurses, and therapists with questionable characters, swollen egos, and poor communication skills, but probably no more than among clergy or college professors. Many of the people who care for us when we are sick are not only highly skilled, but smarter, kinder, and more compassionate than the rest of us. And yet, we are often curiously uncomfortable—not with them personally, but with the power they represent.

Our discomfort with the power of medicine is based on something more than a distrust of physicians and nurses, for the totality of the social power wielded by medicine is both greater and somehow other than the sum of the power possessed and exerted by its individual representatives. What causes us discomfort, I propose, is medicine itself, where "medicine" names not simply a group of professionals trained in a set of practices of caring for persons who are sick, but also an apparently animated social force. We experience this force not simply as more than the sum of its practitioners, their tools, and techniques, as well as the bureaucracy that mediates our access to them, but also as *personified*. In this sense, medicine is not unlike other significant institutions in that it seems to be a kind of supra-human agency that creates its own world. Those who wish to benefit from medicine's power are expected to live in medicine's world and obey its rules, and because that world is sometimes very different from the one to which such hopeful beneficiaries are accustomed, a sense of vulnerability bordering on terror frequently ensues.[31]

Perhaps the best way initially to get a sense of what I mean by this claim is through a consideration of a provocative short story by Lorrie Moore, "People Like That Are the Only People Here: Canonical Babblings in Peed Onk."[32] There Moore tells the story of two relatively sophisticated, middle-class parents who discover that their toddler son has a malignant kidney tumour. As they go through the necessary steps of arranging his medical care, they find themselves pulled into a strange new world. When the parents first learn of their child's illness, they are shocked and overwhelmed by vulnerability. Contemplating the very real possibility of her son's death, the Mother asks, "From where will her own strength come? From some philosophy? From some frigid little philosophy?" She is neither stalwart nor realistic and has trouble with basic concepts, such as the one that says events move in one direction only and do not jump up, turn around, and take themselves back" (219). The Mother is, in other words, very much like most of us, who seldom have or care to take time to contemplate our own fragilities or those of the persons we love.

The only refuge the parents can find from the terror of their situation is in the self-assured expertise of the medical personnel they encounter while seeking treatment for their son's illness, a refuge they share with an ersatz community of others enduring similar trials. "In the end," thinks the Mother, "you suffer alone. But at the beginning you suffer with a whole lot of others. When your child has cancer, you are whisked away to another planet: one of bald-headed little boys. Pediatric Oncology. Peed Onk" (224).

The blunt language here is, no doubt, carefully chosen. For, although Peed Onk initially offers the parents and their new friends a respite from the worst of their terror, they do not experience it as unequivocally benevolent. The Mother soon discovers that Peed Onk is neither a place in a hospital nor an impromptu community of mutual support, but a kind of parallel universe. It is a world with its own language and logic (i.e., its "canonical babblings"), its own ritual practices, and its own social expectations; and those not initiated into its mysteries cannot hope to understand it. "You wash your hands for thirty seconds in antibacterial soap before you are allowed to enter through the swinging doors. You put paper slippers on your shoes. You keep your voice down. A whole place has been designed and decorated for your nightmare. Here is where your nightmare will occur. We've got a room all ready for you" (224). [33]

The taking on of roles in this universe is so parallel that there is no need for personal names. We meet the generically named "Mother," "the Baby," "the Husband," "the Oncologist," and "the Surgeon," while only two patients and one father on Peed Onk retain recognizably personal names. Connections to the "outside world" are bizarre, fragmentary, and alienating: Hospital-provided "courtesy line" calls to friends who recommend having another child as "an heir and a spare;" Christmas carols, bearing an eerie resemblance to the theme from *The Exorcist*, playing over the waiting-room speakers; and fretful nights alone in a tackily appointed lounge named after the ukulele-strumming pop singer Tiny Tim.

The families who occupy the lounge in Peed Onk assume a likeness to each other that exceeds the facts of their common vulnerability and concern for their children's good. Not only do they dress similarly and speak a common, quasi-technical language, they appear to be playing roles, as if they are actors and actresses in an elaborate drama, one that is sometimes tragic, sometimes comic, and always poignant. One of the Mother's friends observes, "Everyone is so friendly here. Is there someone in this place who isn't doing all this airy, scripted optimism—or are people like that the only people here?" (224).

The way the world named Peed Onk pulls on the parents and tries to press them into its mould leaves them—especially the Mother—feeling strangely conflicted. On the one hand she is grateful for the knowledge and skills possessed by its practitioners and the help they give to her son—the alternative, after all, would be that her baby would die, within months or perhaps even weeks. In this sense, she recognizes Peed Onk as a definite good. On the other hand, she senses something is amiss with the "reality" in Peed Onk, something she cannot quite articulate. "It's 'Modern Middle Medicine meets the Modern Middle Family,' says the Husband. 'In the Modern Middle West'" (222). The Mother, an uncertain newcomer to the world, will not accept it. When offered the opportunity by one of her son's physicians, the oncologist, to forego the standard regime of postoperative chemotherapy in favour of a more conservative, albeit experimental, approach that will allow the family to resume life beyond the walls of the hospital, she seizes it with grateful enthusiasm. She is relieved to be free, at least for a time, not so much from the spectre of a therapeutic regimen that would leave her son sick and bald and vulnerable to infection, but from an alien world that controlled her by insisting she be someone she neither was nor was prepared to be.

Moore's story interests me not because it roundly condemns modern medicine (it does not), but because it portrays a conflict—a dis-ease, if you will—analogous to the one Christians should be open to experiencing when they have occasion to engage the world of modern medicine. In that world, God's name is frequently invoked, but seldom in ways that might enable Christians to live more faithfully in the midst of illness. A recent article in *Newsweek* magazine reports on the increasing space given to God in the medical world, noting that more than one half of American medical schools now offer courses dealing with matters of spirituality.[34] In that article, one of the leading physician advocates of a more religiously sensitive medicine suggests that given the "growing body of evidence" that faith can play a significant role in the recovery and maintenance of health, "keeping spirituality out of the clinic is irresponsible."

I am reluctant to dismiss this claim, but I believe it contributes little to the concern to make possible a more faithful Christian use of medicine. To the extent that religious behaviours have been shown empirically to contribute to better health, medicine has enlisted those behaviours in the service of its own projects. Most of the current literature dealing with faith and medicine seems to suggest that spirituality (or religion) should be brought into the world of the clinic and retooled, when and as necessary, to fit and serve the purposes of that world. Christians, in the meantime, have mostly been content to have their tradition so named and enlisted, grateful for the validation, or at least the attention. Yet, this gets matters backwards. It is Christians who ought to be naming medicine, harnessing its power, and bringing it into the service of the way of life of the community called to bear witness to the ongoing work of God in the world.[35] For only as Christians learn properly to name the world and the things in the world can we make proper use of those things. And only as we make proper use of the world can we hope truly to flourish.[36]

By "naming," I mean the act of identifying medicine as belonging in a particular, limited way to the realm of created things. It is my contention that modern medicine may accurately be understood and named as being among, or at least analogous to, what the authors of the New Testament (Paul in particular) call the "Principalities and Powers."[37] To name medicine in this way is not to demonize it, but to harness it as an instrument helpful in the pursuit of the ultimate human good of friendship with God, a good achieved through our learning properly to love, a skill which is in turn learned through the proper worship of the Christian God.

Although the New Testament authors' use of the language of Principalities and Powers is anything but univocal—Walter Wink calls it "imprecise, liquid, interchangeable and unsystematic"[38]—it is thematically consistent enough to serve the purposes of this analysis. The language derives from two distinct and yet overlapping thought worlds. The first and less discussed of these is the world of Greek philosophy, beginning with the Hippocratic philosophers of the fifth century BCE, who spoke of power primarily as a capacity of the human soul. The Greek use of the language of power is taken up in post-biblical Christian tradition in a variety of ways, including the work of the so-called Cappadocian Fathers and Thomas Aquinas, who spoke of the human powers as among the "principles of human acts."[39]

The second, more obvious source of this language is Jewish apocalyptic, which uses the language of power to account for those forces set against the people of God during times of persecution. This apocalyptic use in the New Testament is predicated on the conviction that the world as we experience it day-to-day is, because of its alienation from its Creator and its subsequent corruption, in the process of "passing away." Ultimately, this age—this "present darkness," to use a biblical image—will disappear and will be replaced by the new age of God's reign. In the meantime, it is the task of those gathered together by God to live, to the extent possible, as citizens of the new age. Paul, in 2 Corinthians 5, names this age the "new creation," the members of which are those who confess "Jesus is Lord" by their baptism into his death and resurrection. Those members are to live together in such a way that their life bears witness to God's reign. Lives so lived will in many ways make

Christians appear strange, however, because the world—that is, the part of the creation which refuses to recognize God's reign—remains under the influence of false gods of its own making. As Flannery O'Connor once warned, "You shall know the truth, and the truth shall make you odd."

One way the notion Principalities and Powers functions within the biblical scheme is to describe the seen and unseen, personal and impersonal institutional forces that provide necessary order, or "structure," making possible a common human life during the time preceding the consummation of God's redemptive work.[40] Governments, bureaucracies, and any other highly organized form of human activity may properly be counted among the Powers. John Howard Yoder offers an especially clear account of this way of understanding the biblical usage:

> The most fruitful illustration of the complexity of this language for the modern reader would probably be a meditation on the variety of meanings of the word "structure" as it is currently used in American English. Sometimes it refers to a particular network of persons and agencies able to make decisions or exert pressure, as in the phrase "power structure." When this term is used it may refer to a group of persons who are known or can be found. . . . Other times the "power structure" is not so visible but one is no less sure that it is there. . . . Yet other times "structure" is present only in the mind of the one analyzing it. . . . In all these ways and more we could add, *the concept "structure" functions to point to the patterns or regularities that transcend or precede or condition the individual phenomena we can immediately perceive.*[41]

The biblical authors appear frequently to associate the Powers and Principalities with evil, and even with demonic activity; it is the Powers, Paul says at one point, that were responsible for the death of Jesus (Colossians 2:15). Yet, it is important to note, especially in the context of naming medicine among the Powers, that these same authors regard the Powers neither as absolutely good nor as inherently and irretrievably evil.[42] According to Walter Wink, the New Testament tells the story of the Powers and their role(s) in the world as "a drama in three simultaneous acts: The Powers are good, the Powers are fallen, the Powers will be redeemed."[43] The Powers are good because they are part of God's good creation, both in the sense that they are artifacts of human power and in the sense that they have an existence of their own independent of human agency. The author of the letter to the Colossians includes the Powers among those things owing their existence to the will of Christ, explaining "in him [Christ] all things in heaven and on earth were created, things visible and invisible, whether thrones or dominions or rulers or powers—all things have been created through him and for him" (Colossians 1:16). God has made the Powers to serve God and God's creatures by preserving a relatively just and sometimes peaceable order in the realm of created things. Apart from them, we may assume, things would not function as they should, and we would not be able to discover or pursue goods in common; as John Howard Yoder puts the matter, there is a very real way in which "we cannot live without them."[44]

At the same time, however, neither can we fully "live with" the Powers, at least not as faithful citizens of God's reign.[45] Along with the rest of creation, the Powers are fallen, alienated from the Creator and so from the Creator's intent for them. The origin of this separation is human sin. Disordered human desire—itself a kind of "power"[46]—leads us to be idolaters, to love creatures (including ourselves) after the fashion and with the intensity that only the Creator is properly to be loved. And the Powers, to the extent we can attribute to them something analogous to consciousness, are more than happy to receive our adulation, and so to participate in our fallenness. Says G. B. Caird, "Men had exalted that which was secondary and derivative into a position of absolute worth, and by accepting their worship the rulers had become involved in their sin."[47] The Powers, because of the obvious goods they seem to bestow on human societies, assume in human consciousness a quasi-divine status. This adulation in turn corrupts the proper worship of the God of Israel, Jesus, and the church.[48] Women and men are not simply dependent upon, but bound—enslaved, if you will—by and to the Fallen Powers. As Yoder explains,

> They thereby enslaved man and his history. Man is bound to them; "slavery" is in fact one of the fundamental terms used in the New Testament to describe the lost condition of man outside of Christ. To what is man subject? Precisely to those values and structures which are necessary to life and society, but which have claimed the status of idols and have succeeded in making men serve them as if they were of absolute value.[49]

The influence of the Powers on human consciousness and human life is therefore not necessarily violent; rather, it frequently takes the form of deceit and seduction, of persuading women and men that the Powers control access to and determine human flourishing. And because in our fallen state our understanding of flourishing is forever becoming entangled in the grasp of egotism—that is, injudicious self-love—we are readily so persuaded.[50] As Hendrik Berkhof puts it, "in contrast to the chaos, to which our enmity toward God has condemned us, life under the

Powers is tolerable, even good."[51] In other words, we willingly cooperate with the Powers' pretensions toward divinity because of the apparent short-term benefit our idolatry accrues to us, not the least of which is that the Powers allow and sometimes enable us to continue living. The Powers offer us life; yet, the life they offer may ultimately be at cross-purposes with our well-being because it is predicated on a lie.

The alternative to the idolatry that is bondage to the Powers is the proper worship of God. Lives formed by the proper worship of God do not presume to destroy the Powers, nor to ignore them, but rather to make proper use of them, treating them to the greatest possible extent as having been rendered subject again to God through the life, death, and resurrection of Jesus of Nazareth.[52] According to the author of Colossians, it is through the cross that Jesus "disarmed the rulers and authorities and made a public example of them, triumphing over them in it" (Colossians 2:15). Thus, we find at the very centre of Christianity a kind of irony. In the very act through which the Powers thought they were ridding themselves of the One whose life afforded the profoundest of challenges to their authority, he breaks their idolatrous hold over humanity.

> He "made a public example of them." It is precisely in the crucifixion that the true nature of the Powers has come to light. Previously they were accepted as the most basic and ultimate realities, as the gods of the world. Never had it been perceived, nor could it have been perceived, that this belief was founded on deception. Now that the true God appears on earth in Christ, it becomes apparent that the Powers are inimical to Him, acting not as His instruments but as His adversaries. . . . Obviously, "none of the rulers of this age," who let themselves be worshipped as

> divinities, understood God's wisdom, "for had they known, they would not have crucified the Lord of glory" (1 Corinthians 2:8). Now they are unmasked as false gods by their encounter with very God; they are made a public spectacle.[53]

The Powers' ultimate destiny is to be redeemed by the death and resurrection of Jesus of Nazareth. In the meantime, however, the chief Christian task with respect to the Powers is to resist their seduction, for in spite of their having been defeated, the Powers continue to refuse to assume their proper, subordinate place in the overall scheme of things.[54] Such resistance, however, by no means precludes Christian association with the Powers, which would be inadvisable, much less impossible. "The believer's combat," says Berkhof, "is never to strive *against* the Orders, but rather to battle for God's intention for them, and against their corruption."[55]

For Yoder, this means one thing, namely that "the very existence of the church is her primary task." For that existence "is in itself a proclamation of the Lordship of Christ to the Powers from whose dominion the church has begun to be liberated." Jesus has defeated the Powers, and by its faithful existence as the body of Christ, the Christian community demonstrates that defeat to the world.[56] Berkhof perhaps puts this best when he says, "By her faith and life the Church of Christ labels the dominion of the Powers as *un-self-evident*. She is the turnstile which shuts off all return to the unconscious taken-for-grantedness of the former cultures."[57]

All this leaves open the question of whether medicine can properly be named among the Powers, not to mention describing in any detail how that power might be resisted and faithfully be used in the service of the Christian gospel. Berkhof's remark about the importance of Christians' interrogating and overcoming the "taken-for-grantedness of the former cultures" provides a good place to begin the first task, for it reminds us that medicine, like every other culturally-formed aspect of the yet-to-be redeemed creation within which we exist as Christians, is not simply "there." In spite of its remarkable accomplishments and its generally benevolent face, medicine as we find and experience it remains an artifact of a fallen humanity living in a fallen world. Thus medicine's benefits, while considerable, are not absolute. Christians must therefore use them judiciously.

Who, though, is prepared to confront, rather than acquiesce to, the power of medicine? Where should one begin? Christians would do well to start by noting that medicine primarily functions among the Powers by its occupation of a revered social position, through which it appears to wield nearly sovereign control over life and death. One thing contemporary North Atlantic culture—and this may be true of every culture—has in common with Christianity is its regard for death as an enemy. In contemporary North Atlantic culture, medicine aspires, if not to defeat, then at least to forestall the inevitability of death. Most people living in contemporary North Atlantic culture understand that there are ways in which they or someone they know and love literally owes their lives to modern medicine. It is perfectly appropriate, moreover, to be grateful for this fact. Gratefulness, however, is not the same thing as worship or allegiance, which are perhaps better ways to describe our society's general disposition toward medicine. There is no apparent limit to medicine's ambition to control the circumstances of human life and death by bringing them under human control. Billions of dollars are invested each year in research that has as its ultimate aim the elimination of contingency from the biological circumstances of human existence, and few people seem interested in asking whether or to what extent such an aim is appropriate for creatures of a providential God.

Let me reiterate here one important point: the fundamental interconnectedness of the Powers and the desires and powers of those the Powers hold subject. The medical project of controlling life and defeating death is attractive to us not simply—not even largely—because medicine compels our acceptance, but because a denial of our own mortalities and a desire to be in control and avoid suffering is very near the centre of our own disordered desires. It is certainly the case that the medical industry wants us to believe it wields this kind of power for our good. Think, for example, of how we are bombarded by advertisements for products designed to treat the effects of growing older, conditions like baldness, impotence, and anxiety, advertisements whose message is clearly "you *need* this in order to be happy." Yet, it is also the case that such advertisements succeed because they are so completely consonant with the spirit of our culture, a spirit produced and reproduced by our unchallenged avoidance of our own fragilities. Arthur McGill suggests that the "most crucial task" for this culture is to "create a living world where death seems abnormal and accidental." In such a world,

> Life is so full, so secure, and so rich with possibilities that it gives no hint of death and deprivation. Here we have the first ethical duty imposed by the conviction that death is outside of life and that life is the only good for which we should live. According to this duty, a person must try to live in such a way that he or she does not carry the marks of death, does not exhibit any hint of the failure of life. A person must try to prove by his or her own existence that failure does not belong

> essentially to life. Failure is an accident, a remediable breakdown of the system.[58]

The project by which medicine becomes the chief mediator of the power of death is clearly in some respects a religious one, if by "religious" we mean pertaining to the particular objects of affection around which our lives revolve. Nicholas Lash suggests that contemporary objects of "religious" devotion could include "beliefs and practices protective of . . . things we are too terrified to mention, or of instincts, prejudices and convictions lying at the very heart of who and how we take ourselves and other things to be."[59] In this culture, surely, one such object is the integrity and vigour of our individual bodies. Just so, concludes Arthur McGill,

> If we ask about religion in America, you can see the conclusion which I must draw. The God whom Americans worship as the final and absolute reality is the power of death. Here I do not use the term "god" to designate the divinity revealed in Jesus Christ. I use the word in a more open way, to name what a people believe to be the final, the ultimate reality which controls their lives. Many Americans (notwithstanding their dedicated commitments to the ethics of success and resistance) still believe that death is the ultimate reality that will finally and permanently determine their existence.[60]

It is important to acknowledge, on this side of the grave at least, that death remains a fearsome, indeed an awesome, thing. Few are prepared to welcome, "our sister, bodily death," as St. Francis of Assisi sang on his deathbed. Even Francis required a lifetime of prayer and practice to add "sister death" to his canticle praising God for and through *all* creation, not just the warm and fuzzy bits. Jesus himself wept at the reality of death (before the tomb of Lazarus) as well as the prospect of death (in the Garden of Gethsemane). Moreover, Christians cannot loathe the body—again, God's good creation—or welcome death as merely the liberation from its fleshy prison. Paul, echoing the prophet Isaiah, concludes his extended discussion of the ultimate fate of the body—resurrection—with the cry: "Death has been swallowed up in victory/ Where, O death, is your victory/ Where, O death, is your sting?" (1 Corinthians 15:54-55). Yet, the Christian victory over death is a victory won *through* death, and death seldom is unaccompanied by suffering. The prospect of suffering—perhaps even more than its present reality—inspires fear.

The world in which we live at once "worships" death as ultimate reality and at the same time treats it as practically alien to this life. Because the modern world, in practice if not in word, refuses to trust the God revealed in Christ to save us from death, those sanctioned with the power to preserve life and vigour and to forestall or control death and the suffering associated with it are understood within modern culture to represent god-like power.[61] This is not because these people think of themselves more highly than they ought, but because of the social significance we give to the power they represent. This is how the fallen Powers function; they cooperate with the disordered appetites of those who use and depend upon them, allowing us to see them not as God's instruments, but as gods, period. To a significant extent, they are successful because they promise, in ways that God appears unwilling or incapable, to deliver us from the evil of those contingencies we regard as unhappy or fearsome.[62]

In his seminal work on the Powers and Principalities in the New Testament, G. B. Caird notes that over the course of the biblical narrative, in Judaism and then in Christianity, there is a gradual, nearly imperceptible shift concerning the relationship of God to those events we name as "contingent," especially as they transpire in what we uncritically call the "natural" world. Over the course of this shift, the basic conviction that the God of Abraham and Moses is also "Lord of history" remains constant.[63] As Lord of history, God is depicted in the narrative as generally sovereign over the contingent, both in human nature and in the natural world as such. At the same time, however, the narrative suggests that "There were always recalcitrant elements which refused to be brought within the scope of the divine sovereignty" (57). These "recalcitrant elements" are understood and eventually articulated explicitly in terms of human sin, and give rise to the notion in Judaism and Christianity of both a radical distinction in kind and a breach in relationship between a holy, sovereign Creator and a good, but nonetheless fallen, creation (59). It is the breach in relationship, the alienation of creation from its Creator, which turns contingency into suffering.[64]

This incongruity comes over the course of the New Testament narrative to be depicted increasingly as an eschatological problem, which is to say that there is a developing sense that the unruly remainder, both in human life and the natural world, will be perfected and so fully made subject to God only in the age to come, the consummated kingdom of God. God, who promises a reign free from suffering, controls history and those contingencies within history that cause or allow us to suffer, but that control will be fully manifest only in the age to come. As Caird notes:

> It is worthwhile to notice in passing that the Creation myth plays a large part in the symbolism of Revelation. The crystal sea in heaven represents all that bars man from access to the throne of God. Out

> of the sea rises the beast, which is both the parody and the usurper of God's authority. Like the Red Sea before the Israelites, the heavenly sea parts to allow the martyr throng to pass into the security of the promised land, and having passed they sing the song of Moses and the Lamb. . . . And when the victory of God is complete the heavenly city is revealed, in which there is no more sea.[65]

In the writings of Paul, the New Testament author most concerned to talk about the Powers, Jewish (and Christian) apocalyptic concerns about the eschatological redemption of creation are brought into conversation with popular Greco-Roman thought, which had been heavily influenced by the concerns of Greek philosophy. The great philosophical concern of the Greeks, Caird explains, was to "discover a unity within the manifold facts of experience," a concern that derived from "the realism with which they regarded the phenomena of change and decay" (73)—which is simply to say that they were deeply concerned to find meaning in a world where every living thing ultimately grew old and sick and died. The mystery religions, which Caird believes Paul counts among the Powers, flourished precisely because they professed to offer such meaning.

It is as a voice in this conversation, insists Caird, we should read Paul's ruminations about human suffering and fragility, and especially those dealing with his own weakness and frailty. In his second epistle to the Corinthian church, Paul speaks at some length about such matters, and at one point says that he had been given "a thorn . . . in the flesh, a messenger of Satan to torment me, to keep me from being too elated" (2 Corinthians 12:7). Caird believes that Paul is referring here to a chronic illness, a condition that the Apostle strangely regards at once as incompatible with the ultimate intentions of God and at the same time as a gift from God given to help properly shape his affections (75). "Three times," says Paul, "I appealed to the Lord about this, that it would leave me, but he said to me, 'My grace is sufficient for you, for power is made perfect in weakness'" (2 Corinthians 12:8-9). Paul was able to hold together seemingly incommensurable conclusions about his illness, not because he had some perverse sense that illness was good for him, but because he was convinced that some of the unhappy contingencies that happen to our bodies may have to be borne patiently while we wait for the consummation of God's redemptive work, a work achieved in the cross and resurrection of Jesus of Nazareth (77-78). This patient endurance of suffering, Paul implies, is a fundamental element of a faithful Christian witness to the coming kingdom of God.

Such patient endurance is far from passive. It entails neither an abandonment of hope nor a simplistic projection of hope into the life to come. It is probably not possible to enumerate in advance which must be borne patiently and which attacked and overcome by the instruments of good God has given to us—these are matters of communal discernment that far exceed the scope of this lecture—but we can say that medicine remains among those instruments for which we may be thankful. Yet, to see medicine as an instrument for the promotion of Christian (and so of human) flourishing requires that we learn to see our bodies and the health we enjoy as gifts from God. Only then will we be able to say with the Psalmist that God's "steadfast love is better than life."

Three

Baptism, Communion, and the Body: The Pedagogy of Creaturely Interdependence[66]

We're all in this thing together,
Walkin' the line between faith and fear.
This life won't last forever.
When you cry, I taste the salt of your tears.
—Old Crow Medicine Show

As best I can remember, I was seven or maybe eight years old the first time I was there, probably accompanying my grandfather on his weekly walk to count and salt the cattle and make sure the fences were still up. For a boy that age, it was a hard-earned prize, a walk of an hour or more that demanded the negotiation of steep hills, blackberry brambles, rhododendron thickets, and a half-dozen or so barb wire fences that seemed to have a persistent knack for tearing my shirts and leaving marks on my back. My parents and grandparents called it the Old Home Place. It was the original parcel of my mother's family's farm, the narrow hollow and surrounding steep hills where my mother and her father and grandfather had been born and raised in a rambling old house that had been turned to salvage when I was still in diapers. It is the place where my ancestors are buried. It is the place I most clearly recall in connection to learning who I was, where I had come from, and what kind of things really mattered.

As I grew older, I often walked to the Old Place on my own, the terrain of the hike becoming as familiar to me as my own body. Sometimes I went hunting squirrels, sometimes picking berries, sometimes just for the sake of the walk, but always covering the same well-known ground: Leaving the house, I would walk northeast up the red dirt of Upper Mill Creek Road, cross the creek into the Taylor hollow, and eventually climb up the hill past the pond at the head of the hollow where I sometimes fished for bass and bluegill. From the pasture at the top of the hill, overlooking the Elk River to the northwest, I would turn east and walk through a forest of beech, oak, hickory, and maple, around the southern side of a high knob, emerging from the woods on the spur ridge overlooking the original home site. Even now, from hundreds of miles away, I can see and feel the land's contours. I can hear its sounds and smell its smells: the mud and cattail around the pond and below the cisterns, the rich humus topsoil in the dense hardwood forests, the Hereford cattle grazing on the steep hillside pastures. I can taste the teaberry and mint leaves my grandfather gave me to chew and the paw-paws and blackberries he picked for me to eat. I can see the family cemetery on the point of the ridge, overlooking the hollow below. It is shaded by a massive old oak tree where I used to sit quietly, wondering what it was like to be dead and half-expecting those buried there to speak to me, telling me stories about their lives and mine and the place we shared. I can count the graves, those of my great-great-grandparents and all the generations since, and I can almost hear their voices, carried on the wind.

These memories and experiences are a part of me in a way that exceeds affective subjectivity. They have definitively marked my body and shaped my identity by forging and making evident to me otherwise hidden connections to people and place. As significant parts of the history constituting my life to this point, they have helped make me the person I am. And they have given me a sense of what it means to flourish—to be healthy—as a human being.

Of course, this lecture is not supposed to be about me; it is supposed to be a contribution to our ongoing conversation about worship and bioethics. But that means it is in some sense about human bodies and the health of those bodies, which raises the possibility of connections between my story and questions of bodies and their health. I suspect these connections are far from self-evident to most of the people who "do" bioethics. In the current scientific and political climate, in fact, explicit normative questions about the body and its goods are commonly regarded as matters of speculation or even superstition. Yet, I remain convinced that *all* questions in bioethics are ultimately questions about the nature, destiny, and goods of the human body. This is to say, quite simply, that bioethics is in the final analysis about what bodies are, and what they are for.

This means that we cannot speak at length about the body and its health without speaking as well about matters as far-ranging as theology and agriculture. As Wendell Berry reminds us, "While we live our bodies are moving particles of the earth, joined inextricably both to the soil and to the bodies of other living creatures. It is hardly surprising, then, that there should be some profound resemblances between our treatment of our bodies and our treatment of the earth."[67] Our bodies are not simply contiguous, but also continuous with other bodies and their places on the earth, and this means that nothing less is at stake (in understanding how properly to relate our bodies to the earth and to other creatures) than our health: "by understanding accurately his proper place in Creation, a man may be made whole."[68]

To the extent these assertions seem out of place in a conversation about bioethics, it is due largely to the problematic way the modern moral imagination has conceived the human body. Most standard approaches to bioethics take for granted what most of modern medicine has assumed, which is that the body is somehow distinct from the person associated with it, that it is in some way inhabited by that person, and that it is the private property of that person to dispose of as he or she chooses. Philosophers know this account of the body more or less as *Cartesian*, after the seventh-century French philosopher and mathematician Rene Descartes.[69] Descartes sought to develop a philosophical method built upon a foundation of absolute certainty. Consistent with the scepticism that was fashionable at the time, he engaged in a thought experiment, wherein he systematically doubted everything that could to him conceivably be false. In the end, he believed, he could accept as indisputable only one thing, which was that he, as an individual person, existed as an essentially immaterial thinking thing, a *res cogitans*. His fundamental dictum is well known today, even to non-philosophers: *cogito ergo sum*—"I think, therefore I am."

But if the human subject is an immaterial thinking thing, then what is the human body? Obviously, believed Descartes, the body was something other than the active thinking subject—there was, in other words, an essential *dualism* of person and body. Descartes ultimately said that the body was an artificial, passive extension of the person, a *res extensa* that existed to be manipulated at will by the person inhabiting it. The body was, he suggested, not unlike a *machine*.[70]

Although Cartesian dualism has as a philosophical position died the death of a thousand qualifications, the metaphor of the body as machine and its accompanying dualism has persisted and has probably become the most common way modern people think of themselves and their bodies. Intuitively the Cartesian model has great explanatory power, and it is especially congenial to the body's rendering as an object of scientific investigation.[71] Perhaps most importantly, the machine metaphor is friendly to the modern sociopolitical consciousness, which simultaneously purports to privilege the autonomous will of the individual while conditionally restraining that autonomy in the name of certain kinds of social utility.

The machine metaphor is helpful just to the extent it is true. In some ways and to some extent the human body is like a machine, and I suspect that metaphor has contributed a good deal toward an improved understanding of the human body. This improved understanding, in turn, has produced many medical achievements that are indisputably salutary. Yet, metaphors have limits, and a failure to recognize those limits distorts our knowledge of the things to which our metaphors refer, which in turn distorts the ways we live in the world.[72] This is, I contend, much the case with contemporary medicine, and so with contemporary bioethics. As a branch (or at least an epiphenomenon) of modern medicine, bioethics often has failed critically to account for the limits of the biomedical view of the body, which is decidedly mechanistic. And this failure has meant that bioethics has been unable to say very much about the ways in which modern medicine, because of the limits inherent in the way it imagines the body, has failed or been unable to contribute as fully as it otherwise might to genuine human flourishing.

No one has spoken as clearly and persuasively about the limits of the body-as-machine metaphor as Wendell Berry, who maintains that the machine metaphor is in many respects *unnatural*:

> Of course, the body in most ways is not at all like a machine. Like all living creatures and unlike a machine, the body is not formally self-contained; its boundaries and outlines are not so exactly fixed. The body alone is not, properly speaking, a body.

> Divided from its sources of air, food, drink, clothing, shelter, and companionship, a body is, properly speaking, a cadaver, whereas a machine by itself, shut down or out of fuel, is still a machine.[73]

Yet because we live as if this is not the case, our lives, including the ways we practice healing and caring for the sick, have become distorted.[74] As participants in a radically individualized culture, we think of and treat our bodies as solitary and individual, like machines, and pay relatively little attention to the thousands of ways in which our bodies are connected to other bodies and to our particular places in the world. We forget, ignore, or treat as irrelevant our bodies' surroundings. We discount the idea that our body might have purposes beyond those we individually will for it; purposes, for example, that are based on its relations to bodies or landscapes we have not chosen, or perhaps even inherent in the limits imposed on us by our body's fragility and finitude.[75] Thus, we engage in a kind of ongoing war against limits, that, because of our ignorance of the interdependences that are fundamental to our lives as creatures, expands into a war against each other, against the earth, and ultimately against ourselves and our true flourishing.[76]

Ideally, we should be mindful of the fact that "to speak of the health of an isolated individual is a contradiction in terms,"[77] and that the "grace that is the health of creatures can only be held in common."[78] But because our perception of what constitutes our health is partial and distorted, we fail to attend properly to the ways in which we are increasingly unhealthy. In the United States, medical expenditures on technologically sophisticated therapies that will benefit mainly the rich climb precipitously even as we neglect the welfare of the poor, of children, and of the earth we inhabit.[79] We spend obscene amounts of money preserving the illusion of youth or staving off the death of the well-insured for just a few more days while infant mortality from entirely preventable causes climbs among our poorest neighbours. Our automobiles and power plants spew pollutants while we destroy our watersheds by lopping off the tops of mountains and dumping the remnants into adjacent valleys so we can more cheaply get at the coal beneath the surface. We eat without thinking about what we eat or where it comes from, even as we flush the poisoned topsoil upon which we depend for food down rivers and into oceans that literally are dying to preserve the profits of agribusinesses and chemical companies.

Even though we have managed largely to ignore it, the problem created by our way of life is huge, and the difficulties in trying to overcome it are bound to be legion. And yet, we will not get anywhere close to a satisfying solution if we attempt to mend things quickly through massive, top-down shifts in social or economic policy. Perhaps what we need is to be changed ourselves, to learn to live in, to see, and even to speak differently about the earth and its inhabitants. Such an approach could begin in any number of places. But here I am interested in only one. I propose we learn to live, see, and speak differently with respect to our bodies. Insofar as our speech is dependent upon metaphor, we need to search for and learn to use more truthful metaphors for the human body, and we need to attend to the particular practices that might sustain that speech.

Our search might begin quite simply by considering the ways we learn about bodies in everyday practice. We do not learn about bodies simply by objectively accumulating information about them. Rather, our learning is sensual, and sensually complex. We learn about bodies to a great extent by using our own bodies, and because of this, our learning is by nature intersubjective, meaning the bodies we learn about have significant effects on us as learners.[80] We learn about bodies much in the way we learn about landscapes, the particular places on earth we inhabit. We learn *as* bodies, by touch, taste, smell, and varieties of manipulations and tactile and motor observations that mark and shape both the learning body and the body learned about.

Lovers learn bodies this way, through the accumulated familiarity that comes with the recurrent intertwining of limbs and a thousand mindless caresses. Parents and children learn bodies this way as well, through playful and affectionate gestures, certainly, but also through what Kathleen Norris calls the "quotidian mysteries" of everyday tasks like feeding, bathing, and dressing.[81] Athletes, whose undertakings require extraordinary levels of embodied self-knowledge, develop their skills by testing their bodies and those of their teammates and competitors, acquiring strength and flexibility and learning to use them by exploring and expanding their limits, day after day. And lest I be accused of waxing sentimental, let me point out that students of anatomy—physicians, nurses, and physical therapists, among others—also come to learn about the body first of all by handling bodies, not just those of cadavers, but each others', as well. It is worth noting that such learning begins and always refers back to what anatomists call "landmarks," the body's particular, readily locatable points of reference from which other features may be located and learned. Clearly, the body is, at least as much as it is a machine, a *landscape*, a particular, complex place that is part of and interdependent with its immediate surroundings and, ultimately, all of creation.

Landscapes are, first of all, *particular* places. Although the general laws of the physical and natural sciences are applicable to every landscape, those laws can never approach, let alone exhaust, all there is to be known about any given landscape. Landscapes are particular to themselves and their surroundings and the history of their uses, and they can be known only as they are respectfully explored and inhabited. The boundaries and contours of landscapes are not drawn arbitrarily according to the machinations of political power or economic self-interest, as on a map; rather they emerge, often transiently, through the stories told by those who inhabit and use them.[82]

Landscapes are also, therefore, properly *beloved*. Knowledge of a landscape is never separable from its habitation and use. A place may be known intimately only as it is lived upon and used, and yet it can be inhabited and used well only to the extent that it is loved. To love a particular place is to use it suitably and with the acknowledgement that it has an integrity and a life quite apart from what can be taken from it; to love it is, in other words, to *care* for it. "Land," says Berry, "cannot be properly cared for by people who do not know it intimately, who do not know how to care for it, who are not strongly motivated to care for it, and who cannot afford to care for it."[83] This means that the question of a land's proper use and its integrity is fundamentally historical, in the sense that such questions always appeal to the more basic question of the identity of the people who have longstanding connections to and affection for the land. To have such affection is to desire above all else the land's flourishing, its health. One cannot truly love someone or something one does not know, and such knowledge is by nature historical.[84] The misuse of land by absentee coal and timber companies bears abundant witness to this, as anyone who has lived in or travelled through rural regions like my native West Virginia or my current home in northeastern Pennsylvania can attest.

To love a landscape means, finally, to understand that it is a member of creation, a part of something greater than itself. Its character and proper uses are shaped by its relationship to adjacent landscapes, such that landscapes are never discrete, and the boundaries and transitions between them may be determined only roughly and in part. The health of upland forests and farms affects the health of local watersheds, which in turn affects the health of rivers and oceans and those who depend on them to live. The acknowledgement that a landscape is a member of creation is essentially a claim about how properly to relate to that landscape. Such an acknowledgement is an admission that the place in question is part of something that exists by the grace of divine agency; that it is from God, and a reflection of God's being that ultimately belongs to and is destined to return to God. "The land," God reminded the Israelites, "is mine; with me you are but aliens and tenants. Throughout the land that you hold, you shall provide for the redemption of the land."[85]

The person who realizes that her beloved landscape exists as a member of the entire creation therefore understands that her place, no matter how extensive the history of its belovedness, belongs not to her, but to God. She is its steward, charged for a time with its care. Berry says that this care is best understood as *usufruct*, the right of temporary possession that carries with it the assumption that whatever use is made of a place by its steward will cause it no irreparable damage.[86] One who understands her relationship to her place in this way understands that the "destruction of nature is not just bad stewardship, or stupid economics, or a betrayal of family responsibility; it is the most horrid blasphemy."[87] Love of God and love of creature are thus inseparable, as the writings of both Old and New Testaments remind us repeatedly.

Human bodies are, as I have already said, fundamentally connected to and dependent upon the earth. Beyond and because of that connectedness, moreover, bodies themselves, in their particularity, their belovedness, and their membership within creation, are metaphorical *landscapes of flesh*. In spite of their considerable similarities to each other, bodies are radically particular. Of course it would be silly, much less unhelpful, to discount the value of statistically normative accounts of the body, such as are gained from blood chemistry profiles, pediatric growth charts, and the like. Yet, each body has its own particular history, and only as that history is understood and appreciated in its particularity can a given body be known and cared for. Berry is clearly right when he explains: "The question that *must* be addressed . . . is not how to care for the planet, but how to care for each of the planet's millions of human and natural neighborhoods, each of its millions of small pieces and parcels of land, each of which is in some precious way different from all the others."[88] These human and natural neighbourhoods are constituted by human bodies connected to each other and to their places, whose well-being depends on their being cared for in light of their precious differences.

To care for bodies in their differences, those bodies must be beloved. The one caring must desire the wholeness of the body cared for, not simply in the sense of returning that body to some abstract health as represented by comparison to biostatistical norms, but in the sense of facilitating the progress of its purposeful life in communion with particular other lives.[89] For, as Berry reminds, "no loved one is standardized."

> A body, love insists, is neither a spirit nor a machine; it is not a picture, a diagram, a chart, a graph, an anatomy; it is not an explanation; it is not a law. It is precisely and uniquely what it is. It belongs to the world of love, which is a world of living creatures, natural orders and cycles, many small fragile lights in the dark.[90]

Bodies are loved properly in their particularity, certainly, but only as the love extended toward them accounts for their existence as creatures, who flourish as dependent and interdependent members of God's creation. A body may be loved well only as it is loved within the creaturely boundaries of its fragility and finitude. To love it without respect to these limits is to not love it at all, but to covet it for one's own purposes. The twentieth-century Protestant theologian Karl Barth maintained that human life was properly understood as a gift and a loan from God. To understand life in this way is first of all to understand its origin and continued existence as coming ultimately from God, and not from itself or those who may have a stake in its continuation.[91]

And this means that a body may be properly beloved only in light of its mortality. In this respect health is to be understood "like life in general [as] a temporal and therefore a limited possession."[92] Illness is properly to be resisted, but also to be understood as a harbinger of mortality, which ultimately can be defeated only by God, only through death and resurrection.[93] Acknowledging this as a guiding principle is not fatalism, but "an indispensable form of cultural generosity. It is the one effective way a person has of acknowledging and acting upon the fact of mortality: he will die, others will live after him."[94] Love, Berry explains,

> must confront death, and accept it, and learn from it. Only in confronting death can earthly love learn its true extent, its immortality. Any definition of health that is not silly must include death. The world of love includes death, suffers it, and triumphs over it. The world of efficiency is defeated by death; at death, all its instruments and procedures stop. The world of love continues, and of this grief is the proof.[95]

The question of whether or not it is helpful to think of the body as a landscape of flesh rests on whether such thinking can foster better care of bodies, especially by those whose work is the enterprise we call medicine. One way the landscape metaphor might help those who care for bodies is by encouraging a sense of humility, of the limits of their discipline. Caring for landscapes requires a patient, intimate attention to detail for which expertise, no matter how substantial, is not a substitute. To the extent that a body is like a particular place on earth, the medical professional who seeks to care for it must understand that he is a sort of invited trespasser. If he does not attend adequately to the sympathetic knowledge of those who best know and love that body, he brings to it the capacity to do considerable harm in the name of good. In a short aphoristic essay entitled "Damage," Berry tells a story that nicely illustrates this point.

The story begins with Berry's unambiguous desire to do (what he regarded as) good: "I have a steep wooded hillside that I wanted to be able to pasture occasionally, but it had no permanent water supply."[96] He goes on to tell how he sought to improve his farm by hiring someone to dig a small pond into the hillside. Almost immediately the pond began to fill, and soon enough it was large enough to provide water for a small number of livestock. Yet, for all Berry's good intentions, not to mention his considerable knowledge of and affection for his farm, things did not unfold exactly as he had planned:

> We had an extremely wet fall and winter, with the usual freezing and thawing. The ground grew heavy with water, and soft. The earthwork slumped; a large slice of the wood's floor on the upper side slipped down into the pond.[97]

In reflecting on this damage, which he acknowledges causing, Berry considers how things might have been different. "I was careful," he says, "to get expert advice."

> But this only exemplifies what I already knew. No expert knows everything about every place, not even everything about any place. If one's knowledge of one's whereabouts is insufficient, if one's judgement is unsound, then expert advice is of little use.[98]

The medical stranger who comes to a body wishing to do it good—to improve it—is an expert whose knowledge and skills rightfully garner significant power and esteem. Yet, if she is truly to do good, she must begin by acknowledging the limits of her understanding of the particular body she encounters. She must try to know it not simply as one instantiation of *a* body, but as the particular, beloved body that it is. To do this, she must learn something of its aspirations and affections, its present and past connections to other bodies, and the ways in which it was, is, or has failed to be a beloved body. Most of all, she must respect its sanctity, remembering that its presence to her and indeed to the entire world is as a gift and loan from its Creator. Only by treading lightly over the holy ground that is a landscape of flesh can she hope to count her work on its behalf as genuinely good.[99]

Of course, this is all good and well, but it is one thing to call for a new or different way of talking and thinking about our bodies, and another to animate and sustain such speech and thought as might be requisite to changing our lives. The persistence of the machine metaphor and the highly individualistic political thought with which it has tended to coexist cannot be accounted for simply in terms of a scarcity of knowledge about how things really work. They run deeper than that, and overcoming their many difficulties will take more than the dissemination of information. Change will demand the development of new forms of life, and new forms of life demand deliberate attention to embodied practices. The Christian practices of baptism and communion, rightly understood, have the capacity to serve such ends, for these are the practices by which Christians learn and are reminded that the lives we live, we live in connection—to God, to others, and to the rest of the creation.

The seldom questioned politics of individualism, which sustains the modern affinity for thinking of the body as a machine, along with its concomitant construal of ethics as a matter of balancing the competing rights of self-interested individuals, is for Christians not simply wrongheaded. Rather, it is both consequence and evidence of our self-inflicted estrangement from God, our participation in what Western Christianity since Augustine has called the "fall." As William Cavanaugh explains, "the effect of sin is the very creation of individuals as such, that is, the creation of an ontological distinction between individual and group."[100] The notion that my flourishing and yours may be mutually exclusive, that we are by our very nature competitors for scarce resources who relate only by voluntary association, turns out to be nothing less than acquiescence to sin—and so an abandonment of hope for a peaceable reign of God on earth.

If sin is in some sense manifest in individualism, then liberation from sin—atonement—necessarily overcomes individualism. We are created in the image of a God whose very being is the communion of the persons of the godhead, and our lives are designed to be lives of participation in God and each other and the entirety of creation (which is also in some sense the bearer of the divine image).[101] The brokenness of the fall is separation from God and each other and from the earth upon which we are dependent for our lives, a brokenness that must be overcome if we are to flourish or even to know how to move toward flourishing. Says Cavanaugh, "If sin is scattering into mutual enmity—both between God and humanity and among humans—then redemption will take the form of restoring unity through participation in Christ's Body. . . . The Body of Christ is the locus of mutual participation of God in humanity and humanity in God."[102]

The sacrament of baptism is the practice by which we are made members of Christ's body and participants in the new creation, the practice by which we are offered the possibility of genuine flourishing. Baptism incorporates us into the life of God by bodily uniting us to Jesus in his burial and resurrection. Yet, this is no unmediated individual relationship with a "personal saviour"; in baptism we also are incorporated into each other as members of a common body that in some sense both mediates and displays our relationship to God. The Orthodox theologian John Zizioulas explains that for the baptized, "to be and to be in relation becomes identical." Christian existence is thereby what he calls "ecclesial existence." . . . "Because, in fact, if one should ask, 'How do we see this new biological hypostasis realized in history?' the reply would be, 'In the Church.'"[103]

If baptism is the practice by which women and men are made members of Christ's body, communion is the practice of being re-membered into that body. What the Apostle Paul calls the "world," that aspect of creation that refuses to acknowledge its Creator, is rooted in dismemberment, the Hobbesian vision of a war of all against all. The Eucharist is the means by which the baptized are gathered and re-membered to overcome the world's dismembering energy. The eating together of communion—itself the paradigm of all human eating—is by its very nature a participation not only in the goodness of God, but also of those gathered around the table in each other and in the goodness of creation.

This suggests that to root a proper account of human embodiment and flourishing in the practices of baptism and communion is neither esoteric nor sectarian, for these practices refer not to themselves nor even only to the community God brings into existence through them, but to God's intent for all of creation. John Howard Yoder explains that "the will of God for human socialness as a whole is prefigured by the shape to which the Body of Christ is called. . . . The people of God are called to be today what the world is called to be ultimately."[104] The interdependence and thankfulness displayed in baptism and communion are not simply artifacts of those practices, but the way things are made to be.

Just so, when Paul describes the community he calls the "Body of Christ" in 1 Corinthians 12, he is not simply admonishing the church in Corinth, but also gesturing toward a description of the very fabric of creation. And that description is quite congenial to the metaphor I spoke of earlier, that of comparing the body to a landscape. The celebration of difference, the acceptance and embrace of mutual dependence, and the bearing of each other's sufferings are all ways of being with each other that display to the world God's loving intention for creation.

Four
Burial and the Body: The Pedagogy of Death and Resurrection

> *How do I know whether I shall die easily or with difficulty? I only know that my dying, too, is part of my life.... And then—this is the destination, the limit and the goal for all of us—I shall no longer "be," but I shall be made manifest before the judgement seat of Christ, in and with my whole "being," with all the real good and real evil I have thought, said and done, with all the bitterness I have suffered and all the beauty that I have enjoyed. There I shall only be able to stand as the failure that I doubtless was in all things, but . . . by virtue of his promise, as a* peccator justus. *And as that I shall be able to stand. Then, in the light of grace, all that is now dark will become very clear.*—Karl Barth[105]

I begin this final lecture as I began the first, with a juxtaposition, this one not of words, but of images, either or both of which you may find familiar. The first image is of the gathered faithful on Ash Wednesday, which signals for most of Christianity the beginning of the forty-day penitential season named Lent. At the centre of the Ash Wednesday liturgy is the ritual of the imposition of ashes. The ashes of the burned palm fronds from the previous year's Palm Sunday celebration are mixed with oil or water and imposed in the form of a cross upon the foreheads of the membership. And every year, if the community is faithful to its tradition, every member receives the same earnest reminder, as the minister draws their faces close to her own after the imposition and whispers in their ears: "Remember you are dust, and to dust you shall return." The movement of the body of Christ toward the greatest of Christian celebrations begins with the indispensable *aide memoire* that our lives are circumscribed by death; that all of us, rich and poor, female and male, young and old, vital and infirm, are fated to be rendered into the basic elements from which our bodies derive.

The second image is a very different one. At any given time, in any given hospital in the United States, the bodies of a significant number of the patients in the Intensive Care Unit(s) are being sustained with virtually no hope of recovery by the most sophisticated and expensive technology available. Machines and medications, sometimes in vast array, balance their blood chemistries and fluid dynamics. Often, these interventions work so well as to give these women and men the statistical appearance of health. Yet they are far from healthy. They will linger there, for days, weeks, or sometimes even months, because someone—usually a family member, but sometimes a physician or the patient him or herself—refuses to admit that this person's life is drawing to its end and that the technology being employed is only prolonging his or her dying. They remain there because someone—they or those speaking on their behalf or those charged with their care—has not heard, or does not believe, or hopes against the truthfulness of the Ash Wednesday admonition: "Remember you are dust, and to dust you shall return."

This scenario is problematic for a host of reasons: because of the inordinate burdens it imposes; the resources it consumes; and especially the unspoken illusion it helps perpetuate, that somewhere, somehow, if we can just be patient and learn a bit more and get the technology right, we may yet defeat the enemy named death. This illusion does not have its roots in the presumptuous ambitions of contemporary medicine and biotechnology, for medicine and biotechnology, after all, are to significant extent artifacts of culture. As I have sometimes said, we get the medicine and the doctors we ask for, even when we are unaware of our asking. Nor is the illusion founded upon the cultural aspirations of what we often call "modernity," although the modern turn, with its resolve to make humanity the measure of all things and its subsequent worship of freedom and efficiency, certainly has played a significant role in its taking so solid a foothold in our imaginations. Rather, the illusion that death may be escaped—along with the unquenchable desire to escape it—begins as but the clearest among many expressions of the human estrangement from God. Faithful discipleship demands this illusion be overcome.

In that most quotable of movies, *The Princess Bride*, the character Wesley reproves the six-fingered villain, who has just promised not to harm him, but obviously intends his death, "We are men of action. Lies do not become us." And so they do not. We ought to speak the truth, for the truth, as Jesus reminds us, will set us free. But to speak the truth we must first know it, and it is not readily evident that many of us really know the truth where our own deaths are concerned. Of course, to a person everyone of sound mind readily admits to his or her own mortality; and yet this admission is likely to be for most of us merely an abstraction, something to which we assent, begrudgingly, before hurrying back to what Ernest Becker called our own personal "projects of *causa sui*;" that is, our projects of self creation.[106] These projects (about which I will say more momentarily) struggle against and, more often than not, purge from our consciousnesses the truth of our deaths. They are the means by which we obscure from ourselves the unhappy reality that we are finite, mortal beings. They are edifices unwittingly constructed to hold terror at bay.[107]

Leo Tolstoy's short story "The Death of Ivan Ilych" offers us a view of this struggle and its difficult resolution in the life of one man, a fictional nineteenth-century Russian bureaucrat named Ivan Ilych. In what has probably become the story's most-quoted passage, Tolstoy grants us access to Ivan Ilych's private consideration that the sickness from which he is suffering will be the sickness that ends his life. In spite of the fact that his physicians have so far not been forthcoming about his condition:

> In the depth of his heart he knew he was dying, but not only was he not accustomed to the thought, he simply did not and could not grasp it.
>
> The syllogism he had learned from Keitzewetter's Logic: "Caius is a man, men are mortal, therefore Caius is mortal," had always seemed to him correct as applied to Caius, but certainly not as applied to himself. That Caius—man in the abstract—was mortal, was perfectly correct, but he was not Caius, not an abstract man, but a creature quite, quite separate from all others. . . . "Caius really was mortal, and it was right for him to die; but for me, little Vanya, Ivan Ilych, with all my thoughts and emotions, it's altogether a different matter. It cannot be that I ought to die. That would be too terrible."[108]

Tolstoy's protagonist regards his inability to come to terms with death not simply as an aporia, but as an injustice, a rending of the fabric of his universe:

> "If I had to die like Caius I should have known it was so. An inner voice would have told me so, but

> there was nothing of the sort in me and I and all my friends felt that our case was quite different from that of Caius. And now here it is!" he said to himself. "It can't be. It's impossible! But here it is. How is this? How is one to understand it?"[109]

Two things seem especially remarkable about this passage. The first is Ivan Ilych's belief that he should somehow have known this was coming; that in a just world, he would have had the time, the resources, and the strength to prepare—that he could, if you will, have overcome or at least tamed the monster death. The second thing to note is that here Ivan Ilych begins for the first time to entertain the possibility that his inability to make some peace with his death is a symptom of a cultural sickness. In saying that he thought that "*I and all my friends* felt that our case was quite different from that of Caius,"[110] Ivan Ilych is numbering himself among a somewhat larger community of persons likewise deceived. Thus the story is not simply about one man's difficulty wrestling with the truth about his dying, for Ivan Ilych's difficulty coming to terms with his mortality is not simply a character flaw peculiar to Ivan Ilych, flawed though he may have been. Rather, that difficulty is part of the brokenness Tolstoy understood to be characteristic of the human predicament and the ways that brokenness is veiled by certain forms of common life. When sin is universally normative, then it becomes very difficult to name as sin.

In another scene from the story, the setting of which is Ilych's wake, one of his friends and colleagues has come to the home of the deceased to pay his respects. Over the course of his time there, and in the midst of the formal pleasantries typical of such occasions, Peter Ivanovich eventually and quite reluctantly makes his way to Ivan Ilych's coffin:

> The expression on the face said that what was necessary had been accomplished, and accomplished rightly. Besides this, there was in that expression a reproach and a warning to the living. This warning seemed to Peter Ivanovich out of place, or at least not applicable to him. He felt a certain discomfort and so hurriedly crossed himself once more and turned and went out the door—too hurriedly and too regardless of propriety, as he himself was aware.[111]

It is worth noting that Peter Ivanovich goes straight from his friend's wake to join another group of friends for cards and gossip. Just so, Tolstoy wants us to see ourselves, if not in Ivan Ilych, then in Peter Ivanovich. He wants us to consider the ways we wage an ongoing battle of avoidance against the certainty of death we carry around in our bodies, for nearly all of us fight to stave off the terror that threatens to besiege us. And because our principal weapon in that struggle is some form or another of self-deception, even the smallest victory we achieve is bound to be Pyrrhic. The great tragedy (or should I say near tragedy?) of Ivan Ilych's life is its immersion in the everyday self-deception that masqueraded as the ordinary life of a successful, ambitious man of his time. In the story's most telling words, Tolstoy writes that "Ivan Ilych's life had been most simple and most ordinary and therefore most terrible."[112]

The cultural anthropologist Ernest Becker believed that such total self-immersion in culturally normative expectation is the primary means by which most of us flee the terror created by knowing we will die.[113] That terror is expelled or at least controlled, he argues, by placing one's "life project" in the hands of cultural expectations, the achievement of which could nonetheless be regarded as individual success:

> What we will see is that man cuts out for himself a manageable world; he throws himself into action uncritically, unthinkingly. He accepts the cultural programming that turns his nose where it is supposed to look; he doesn't bite the world off in one piece as a giant would, but in small manageable pieces, as a beaver does. He uses all kinds of techniques, which we call "character defenses": he learns not to expose himself, not to stand out; he learns to embed himself in other-power, both of concrete persons and of things and cultural commands; the result is that he comes to exist in the imagined infallibility of the world around him. He doesn't have to have fears when his feet are solidly mired and his life is mapped out in a ready-made maze.[114]

To immerse oneself uncritically in the enticements and demands of mass culture is to participate in the cult of the successful self. It is to cultivate a kind of narcissism that allows and even encourages a denial of the limits inherent in embodied finitude. The idea here seems to be that one can achieve a kind of immortality insofar as one can be seen as the author of a successful life project. Wendell Berry gives us a provocative depiction of this way of life in the opening lines of his wonderful poem, "The Mad Farmer Liberation Front," where he writes:

> Love the quick profit, the annual raise,
> vacation with pay. Want more
> of everything ready-made. Be afraid
> to know your neighbors and to die.
> And you will have a window in your head.
> Not even your future will be a mystery
> any more. Your mind will be punched in a card

and shut away in a little drawer.
When they want you to buy something
they will call you. When they want you
to die for profit they will let you know.[115]

In the end, to live this way is tacitly to deny or simply to forget that one is a creature.[116] Knowing oneself as a creature is more than a matter of assent—more than saying, "Yes, someone else made me, now let's get on with it, I have things to do." Rather, it is to engage in the difficult and costly work of confronting the terror that comes from knowing one is not and cannot be in control. In so doing, one confronts the possibility of despair, of course, but also the possibility of hope, for to be a creature is to stand in awe before one's Creator. Says Becker:

> And so the arrival at new possibility, at new reality, by the destruction of the self through facing up to the anxiety of terror of existence. The self must be destroyed, brought down to nothing, in order for self-transcendence to begin. Then the self can begin to relate itself to powers beyond itself. It has to thrash around in its finitude, it has to "die" in order to question that finitude. To what? Kierkegaard answers: to infinitude, to absolute transcendence to the Ultimate Power of Creation which made finite creatures.[117]

Certainly one can argue with whether this process is necessarily as existentially dramatic as Becker or Kierkegaard indicates. Indeed, I think it does not need to be. Nonetheless, some form of confrontation with one's creatureliness—one's bodiliness, one's finitude, one's mortality—is requisite to faithfulness. "One goes through it all," says Becker, "to arrive at faith, the faith that one's creatureliness has some meaning to a Creator; that despite one's true insignificance, weakness, death, one's existence has meaning in some ultimate sense . . . ."[118]

The call to abandon the pretensions of mass culture and turn in faith toward God is for me evocative of the opening lines of Dante's *Divine Comedy*, in which the poet says:

> In the middle of life's journey, I went astray
> from the straight road and woke to find myself
> lost in a dark wood. How shall I say
> what wood that was! I never saw so drear,
> so rank, so arduous a wilderness!
> Its very memory gives shape to fear.[119]

These inexhaustibly suggestive lines call our attention not to the fact that we are lost, but that most of us have no idea we are lost, because we are happily sleepwalking in pursuit of false gods of our own making. Dante's admonition is to stop what we are doing, to wake up, and to allow ourselves to be confronted by the simple, ordinary, terribleness of everyday life, for only then may we see beyond ourselves. As Dante continues in lines 10-21 of that first Canto:

> How I came to [that place] I cannot rightly say,
> so drugged and loose with sleep had I become
> when I first wandered there from the True Way.
> But at the far end of that valley of evil
> whose maze had sapped my very heart with fear
> I found myself before a little hill,
> and lifted up my eyes. Its shoulders glowed
> already with the sweet rays of that planet
> whose virtue leads men straight on every road,
> and the shining strengthened me against the fright
> whose agony had wracked the lake of my heart

through all the terrors of that piteous night.

Here we are brought to the limits of the existentialist and psychoanalytic perspectives; here we see why Kierkegaard remarked that "So soon as psychology has finished with dread, it has nothing to do but give it over to dogmatics."[120] For it is axiomatic for Christians that "the planet whose virtue leads men straight on every road" (one of Dante's many stunning locutions for God) graciously reveals itself to us *and* enables our movement toward it. Dante has his first glimpse of God in the first twenty lines of a poem that goes on for more than 13,000 lines, and his first attempts to reach God directly are thwarted, in large part by his own incontinence. His partial and provisional achievement of the beatific vision comes only at the poem's end, and only after a long and arduous process of re-formation. The message here is clear: Dante wants us to see that we, too, are in need of re-formation if we wish to receive beatitude. We must learn, insofar as it is possible, to live and to die well, and for this learning we are dependent upon God.

And this brings us back to our starting place, the Ash Wednesday admonition to remember that we come from and are destined to return to the dust of the earth. Not many of us—certainly I am not—are prepared for such remembering apart from our formation by practices that help us see ourselves as we ought. A case can be made for any of several such practices, but here I want to speak briefly about only one, the practice of the Christian funeral, which I understand as the Christian pedagogy of death and resurrection.

In his remarkable book *The Dominion of the Dead*, Robert Pogue Harrison argues that since the Neolithic era, a practical awareness of our connectedness—to the earth and to each other—has marked us as human. The very word "human," he points out, shares a root with the Latin *humus*, earth. Thus, he says, human cultural memory has been sustained for as many as twelve thousand years by our practices of cultivating the earth to feed ourselves and burying our dead and marking their places of burial. These practices and all they entail are the things that remind us of our connections to the earth and to human generations past and future.

As these practices, which remained relatively constant for millennia, have eroded, so has our cultural memory. When I tell my students that I grew up around the graves of my great-great grandparents and all the succeeding generations, all contained within the same small hilltop parcel, they respond with incredulity or, almost as often, the same vague bemusement with which they regard my insistence that the Vietnam War really happened or that Saint Augustine was a real historical figure. And they are even more disbelieving when I talk about the smell of fertile soil or the taste of produce fresh from the garden or the experience of hog killing; for them, food comes from the grocery store or, more often, the fast food restaurant. "When the 'from' of the things we consume becomes not only remote but essentially unreal," says Harrison, "the world we live in draws a veil over the earth we live on, a veil that obscures not only the source of our foodstuffs but also the source of our relation to the earth, namely our death. For the earth is both our *unde*, or 'from,' as well as our *quo*, or 'whereto.'"[121]

The severing and obscuring of our relationships with the earth, Harrison says, are symptoms of our flight from mortality. And yet,

> No amount of emancipation, be it through mechanized food production, technological innovation, or genetic engineering, can absolve us

> from the humus that makes up the "substance" of humanity, regardless of whether biomedical science will eventually find ways to prolong human life indefinitely. Endless prolongation of life does not amount to absolution. Mortality is absolved only by dying. The destruction of place that is occurring almost everywhere at present, and that has been occurring for some time now, is linked in part to an anxious and even frenzied flight from death. We are running away from ourselves, not so much in the sense that we are abandoning our traditional homelands, but in the sense that we are forsaking or destroying the places where our dying can make itself at home.[122]

Just so, it will be a rediscovery and embrace of our connectedness, to the earth and to each other across time, which will allow us once more to approach death and to begin again to discuss the possibility of a "good" death. A return to traditional funerary practices that place us in relation to the earth and to generations past and future might help us rediscover these connections. But this will require an intentional determination to resist the broad cultural trend toward the removal of these practices from the purview of family, community, and church and their attendant placement in the hands of an industry seemingly committed to enhancing our self-deception by making death invisible or surreal or both.

But this resistance cannot be simply a matter of will; rather, it must be a response to God's grace. Christians can resist the funerary practices of modern mass culture and the denial of death represented by those practices because the meaning of death and burial are transformed by the resurrection of Jesus from the dead. The empty tomb of Jesus of Nazareth, says Harrison, changes the traditional relation of the living and the dead, such that: "Grief, mourning, and remembrance, once the dominant modalities of relating to the dead, now become preludes to hope, expectation, and anticipation. One might say that Christianity rendered the souls of the living and those of the dead continuous in a new way, as if the living soul were already dead, while the dead soul, in the very same sense, were still alive."[123]

Note that Harrison does not say that the resurrection makes death any less painful, any less fearsome, any less inscrutable, or any less real. The emphasis is on the way Jesus' resurrection establishes a new continuity of life and death, offering to the living an identity based in part on their relation to the dead. This claim is reminiscent of Paul's account of baptism in Romans, chapter 6. Baptism, he writes there, unites the participant to Christ in his death, burial, and resurrection. Thus baptism is both a death and an anticipation of a new life through and beyond death. "For if we have been united with him in a death like his," says Paul, "we will certainly be united to him in a resurrection like his."[124]

But this anticipatory death and resurrection does not call Christians away from this life, for the new creation is not radically discontinuous with the old. Our bodies and the earth upon which they depend (and to which they will return) are not rendered *un*important, but radically more so. For in the resurrection and ascension of Jesus and the subsequent coming of the Holy Spirit, God is radically present, in our bodies, in the body (of Christ), and in the materiality of the sacraments that nourish us. Thus the entirety of material creation participates in the sacredness of God. Says Harrison:

> It is hardly an exaggeration to say that, theologically speaking, the whole earth becomes, for the person of

> faith, the empty tomb of Easter morning—a place rendered sacred, not because it is swollen with the bones of those who died, but because its law of death has been overturned by Christ during his residence in the tomb. . . . Jesus' corpse . . . has become the new mystical body of Christ. In its resurrected and sacramental plenitude, it does not receive but now dispenses anointment, blessing the earth and giving new life to its otherwise dead matter. In and through that resurrected body, the earth and the cosmos are transfigured. . . . Filled with the promise of new life, the earth as a whole becomes not a conglomerate of places, but *one* new place: the place of Easter morning.[125]

This does not mean that the earth is flattened, such that every place is any place and every body any body. Rather, it means that all of the earth (every particular place) and every body in it (every particular body) is potentially sanctified, potentially a sign, in their particularity, of God's reign. Because baptism is offered to all, without respect to age, gender, class, ethnicity, or nationality,[126] and because Eucharist is offered to all of the baptized, these are universal participations in the death, burial, and resurrection of Christ. Yet, the sheer materiality of these sacraments means they cannot be celebrated except locally, by particular people in particular places. For regardless of how one understands the particular mode of God's presence to these practices, all Christians agree that presence coincides with some form or another of particular human bodies gathered in a place to engage in the activities of washing, eating, and drinking. The waters of baptism are consecrated, but they are waters from (however remotely) particular streams draining particular watersheds, both of which are beloved by particular people. Similarly, the bread and wine are consecrated as signs of the body and blood of Jesus, but they remain bread made from grain and wine from grapes from particular fields and vineyards, nurtured and harvested by particular farmers with particular attachments to those places. Thus the universality (or catholicity) of the church includes, without obliterating, its local particularity. This duality is seen most clearly in the historical Eucharistic prayers, during which God's presence is invoked not simply upon the gifts of bread and wine, but also upon the gathered faithful, the diachronic communion of saints, and the whole world. The commemoration of the death and resurrection of Christ celebrated in communion thus becomes a commemoration, that is, a bringing together, of the gathered, the deceased, and ultimately of all creation.[127]

This accounts for the distinctly baptismal and eucharistic character of traditional funeral liturgies in most strands of Christian tradition. Just as baptism and Eucharist are both celebrations of Christian participation in the death, burial and resurrection of Jesus, Christian funeral liturgies often include or refer explicitly to baptism and Eucharist. As in baptism and Eucharist the participant is united to Jesus in his death and resurrection, the commemoration of the deceased in a Christian funeral is a declaration that those gathered, by virtue of their sharing a baptism, and by virtue of their eating together, share an eschatological future.[128] They share that future with each other; with the deceased around whose body they gather; with the dead in Christ from every generation; and with Jesus himself.

Lest you think I am being too liturgically formal, or too theoretically abstract, or that I am simply suggesting that more proper funerals, better attention to baptismal rituals, and more frequent communion will overcome our difficulties with death, let me offer as an illustration to the contrary a story with a decidedly *non*-liturgical bent. Some of you might find it familiar; it is from one of the short stories of Wendell Berry, entitled "Fidelity."[129] Like all of Berry's fiction, it is set in the Kentucky farming community of Port William, inhabited by a familiar cast of characters Berry (and his readers) refer to as "the Membership." In this particular story we read of the death of one of the community's stalwarts, an old man named Burley Coulter.

At the story's beginning we see Burley, who is in a hospital in the distant city of Louisville, through the minds' eyes of his son Danny and his daughter-in-law, Lyda, who lay sleeplessly, "disturbed beyond the power to think by the thought of the old man who was lying slack and still in the mechanical room, in the merciless light, with a tube in his nose and a tube needled into his arm and a tube draining his bladder into a plastic bag that hung beneath the bed."[130]

It seems clear to his family that Burley is dying. Yet it is not his death keeping those who love him awake at night, but the circumstances of his dying—the manner in which he is being made to die. He has been cut off from those with whom he has shared his life, even though they are in his hospital room every night, "offering themselves where they could not be received. They were brought back as if by mere habit into the presence of a life that had once included them and now did not, for it was a life that, so far as they could see, no longer included even itself" (108).

What is compelling about the story "Fidelity" is its account of how Burley has come to be separated from the people and place whose lives included his own, and, more importantly, how he comes to be returned to them. Both his going and his coming back are the result of the connections Burley has forged over the years with friends and family and place. When Burley became ill, the women and men who loved him took him, perhaps against their better judgement, to the doctor "because they wanted to do more for him than they could do, and they could think of nothing else" (110). Yet in spite of the best efforts of the physicians and nurses in

Louisville, he continued to decline. When he lapsed into a coma, his physicians remained stubbornly optimistic, apparently convinced of his eventual recovery. Soon, however, his family sees that recovery is not likely.

> When they returned on yet another visit and found the old body still as it had been, a mere passive addition to the complicated machines that kept it minimally alive, they saw finally that in their attempt to help they had not helped but only complicated his disease beyond their power to help. And they thought with regret of the time when the thing that was wrong with him had been simply unknown, and there had been only it and him and him and them in the place they had known together. Loving him, wanting to help him, they had given him over to "the best of modern medical care"—which meant, as they now saw, that they had abandoned him.[131]

The point here is not that medicine and medical technology are bad, but that medicine and medical technology are *for* something. They exist not for their own sake, but are at their best when they are in the service of, and contributing to, human flourishing. And human flourishing does not simply include, but requires, membership in a community of friends who love one another. When technology removes us from such communities, especially when there is little possibility that it will be able to return us to them, it is by definition no longer contributing to our flourishing. Some of the Port William membership, those who have been the closest members of the life that has been Burley Coulter, have made a mistake, and they respond to it now by going back and making it right, by overcoming the wound that is the separation of the life of one of their own from their life together.

In the middle of the night, Danny goes to the hospital and takes Burley away, disconnecting the tubes joining him to the world of the hospital and removing him secretly to another world altogether, the world of the membership, the world both men know and love. In an old barn up a long since overgrown hollow, Danny stays with the old man, talking to him, comforting him and assuring him as he slips away into death, "You're all right. You don't have to worry about a thing" (116). Carefully, Danny crafts a grave beneath a tree beside the barn, lining it with flat stones, and reminding himself all the time, "These are the last things now. Everything that happens now happens for the last time in his life" (133). And finally, when Burley has taken his last breath, Danny buries him, speaking aloud a prayer at once simple and full of meaning, "Be with him, as he has been with us" (169). When asked later to account for his actions, Danny says only, "I had an account to settle with one of my creditors" (189).

Berry's poem, "Mad Farmer Liberation Front," from which I quoted above, ends with the obscure admonition: "practice resurrection." In an admittedly attenuated form, practicing resurrection is what Danny is doing in burying Burley in the place on earth they had shared as father and son. Practicing resurrection is what Christians do when they gather, whether to celebrate a baptism, to eat the Lord's Supper, or to celebrate the life of one of their own who has died. This, finally, is at the centre of what it means to be Christian: to be sick as a Christian, to suffer as a Christian, to be present as a Christian to those who are sick or suffering, and, finally, to approach death as a Christian. It is to practice resurrection, knowing that being Christian is a matter of "being with." It is to know that we belong, in sickness and in health, in flourishing and in suffering, and finally in death to the earth, to each other, and to God. It is to know that our stewardship of each other's lives and our stewardship of the earth makes every one of us debtors, to the earth and to every other one, because in every aspect of our lives and then in our deaths, we remain members of God. It means that we must take time and to make room, understanding that being sick and, especially being with those who are sick or suffering, does not take time away from life. Rather, these are the things of life itself, for these are things transformed by the hope of resurrection.

Notes

[1] Saint Basil the Great, "The Long Rules," in *Saint Basil: Ascetical Works,* trans. M. Monica Wagner (New York: Fathers of the Church, 1950), 224.
[2] Wendell Berry, "Healing," in *What Are People For?* (New York: North Point Press, 1990), 9.
[3] Genesis 3:8-19.
[4] I take the idea of worship as the orientation of life (toward God) from Daniel Hardy, "Worship as the Orientation of Life to God," in *Ex Auditu* 8: 2 (1992): 55-71.
[5] Nicholas Lash, "Reality, Wisdom and Delight," in *The Beginning and the End of "Religion"* (New York: Cambridge University Press, 1996), 49-50.
[6] Ibid., 50-51.
[7] Martin Luther, "The Large Catechism," in *Triglot Concordia: The Symbolical Books of the Evangelical Lutheran Church* (St. Louis: Concordia Publishing House, 1921), found at http://www.ccel.org.
[8] Ibid.
[9] Lash, "The Beginning and the End of 'Religion'?" in *The Beginning and the End of "Religion,"* 21.
[10] Wendell Berry, "The Body and the Earth," in *Recollected Essays 1965-1980* (New York: North Point Press, 1998), 270.
[11] Ibid., 271.
[12] Ibid., 276.
[13] Hardy, "Worship as the Orientation of Life to God," 62-64.
[14] Wendell Berry, "Health as Membership," in *Another Turn of the Crank* (Washington: Counterpoint, 1995), 86-109.
[15] Basil, "The Long Rules," 330.
[16] For an extended consideration of these matters, see Joel Shuman and Keith Meador, *Heal Thyself: Spirituality, Medicine and the Distortion of Christianity* (New York: Oxford, 2003).
[17] Basil, "The Long Rules," 331.

[18] Here see Hans Frei, *The Eclipse of Biblical Narrative* (New Haven: Yale University Press, 1974), 3; 130. Cf. Lash, *The Beginning and the End of "Religion,"* 148.
[19] Gerald McKenny, *To Relieve the Human Condition* (New York: SUNY Press, 1997).
[20] Michel de Certeau, "Believing and Making People Believe," in Graham Ward, ed., *The de Certeau Reader* (Oxford: Basil Blackwell, 2000), 125. Quoted in William Cavanaugh, *Theopolitical Imagination* (New York: Continuum, 2002), 79.
[21] Flannery O'Connor, *The Habit of Being*, ed. Sally Fitzgerald (New York: Farrar, Strauss, and Giroux, 1979), 100.
[22] Flannery O'Connor, "Revelation," in *The Complete Stories of Flannery O'Connor* (New York: Farrar, Straus and Giroux, 1971), 508.
[23] Revelation 21:3-4.
[24] Forms of this lecture have been previously published in my book with Brian Volck, *Reclaiming the Body: Christians and the Faithful Use of Modern Medicine* (Grand Rapids: Brazos, 2006), and in *Ex Auditu* 21 (2005): 52-66.
[25] One could just as well say that power is the capacity of an agent to have an effect on a patient, or that power is the capacity to have an effect, period (which allows for the possibility that power is neither always explicitly intentional nor directed toward any one concrete other). I am grateful to Alex Sider and Trecy Lysaught for helping me refine my understanding of power.
[26] I think here especially of the work of Michel Foucault.
[27] I will leave unanswered the very interesting question of whether modern liberalism itself forms a trajectory toward a kind of totalitarianism.
[28] For a more extended discussion of some of these accounts of power, especially as it pertains to medicine, see Joel Shuman, *The Body of Compassion: Ethics, Medicine and the Church* (Boulder: Westview, 1999), 28-44.
[29] Francis Bacon's adage, "Knowledge Is Power," (*Meditationes Sacrae*, 1597) implies power to act, to change things. Bacon makes this explicit through his *Great Instauration*, while maintaining that such action must be motivated by charity. If by "knowledge" we

mean no more than a collection of facts divorced from action, what power such knowledge yields, however well-intentioned, seems suspect. A mother who knew all about her child's needs yet never responded to them might be considered neglectful at best.

[30] See, for example, Michel Foucault, *The Birth of the Clinic: An Archaeology of Medical Perception* (New York: Vintage, 1975); and Howard Brody, *The Healer's Power* (New Haven: Yale University Press, 1992).

[31] This is not to deny the probable prior existence of vulnerability and terror created by the very fact of the illness bringing persons into contact with medicine in the first place, which is often exacerbated by the aforementioned.

[32] Lorrie Moore, *Birds of America* (New York: Picador USA, 1999).

[33] The ritualized, quasi-religious behaviours of the modern hospital further endow medicine with an aura of power and the promise of "salvation" from illness and pain. As we noted in the previous chapter, Stanley Hauerwas advises, ". . . if you want to have a sense of what medieval Catholicism felt like, become part of a major medical center. You will discover there an exemplification of the Byzantine politics often associated with the papacy in its heyday." From *Dispatches from the Front* (Durham: Duke University Press, 1994), 27.

[34] Claudia Kalb, "Faith & Healing," *Newsweek*, 12 November 2003, 47.

[35]Bringing religious practices into the service of something less than God and God's gathered people—a transgression the Bible names idolatry—has a long, disastrous history Christians would do well to recall: Holy War, pogroms against Jews, colonialism, racism, and even the capitulation of liberal Christianity to the Nazis by the so-called "German Christians" are all representative of this legacy.

[36] I take it to be a significant part of the message of the prophets of the Old Testament and of Jesus of Nazareth that true human flourishing requires the proper worship of God, a worship entailing a commitment to a particular form of common life that makes visible God's love for the creation.

[37] For this way of thinking about medicine I am indebted especially to Ross Smillie, who suggested it to me some years ago in a seminar in medical ethics at Duke University.
[38] Walter Wink, *Naming the Powers: The Language of Power in the New Testament* (Philadelphia: Fortress, 1984), 9.
[39] Here I am indebted to Alex Sider, and especially to his unpublished paper, "Who Durst Defy the Omnipotent to Arms."
[40] Hendrik Berkhof suggests that the significance of Paul's speaking of fallen angelic and demonic Powers in the same passages as he speaks of institutional and political Powers is that the Apostle wants to emphasize what these entities have in common, namely, "that these Powers condition earthly life." Hendrik Berkhof, *Christ and the Powers* (Scottdale: Herald Press, 1977), 19.
[41] John Howard Yoder, *The Politics of Jesus* (Grand Rapids: Eerdmans, 1972), 139-140, emphasis mine.
[42] An excellent account of the historic origins of the New Testament language of Principalities and Powers is offered by G. B. Caird, *Principalities and Powers: A Study in Pauline Theology* (Eugene: Wipf & Stock, 2003).
[43] Walter Wink, *Engaging the Powers: Discernment and Resistance in a World of Domination* (Philadelphia: Fortress, 1992), 65.
[44] Yoder, *Politics of Jesus*, 146.
[45] Ibid.
[46] Again, I am grateful to Alex Sider for directing my attention to the complex history of Christian usages of the language of "power." Although a detailed discussion of that history is beyond the scope of this essay, it is worth noting that the language disappears from Christian usage at the end of the Apostolic period, re-emerging in the late fourth century in the work of the Cappadocian Fathers, who use it primarily to refer not to world powers, but to the powers of the human soul. Only in the twentieth century does the explicitly sociopolitical usage of the language re-emerge. As I suggest here, however, the two usages are properly interconnected, in the sense that the powers maintain their status as

quasi-divine by virtue of their willingness to satisfy (as well as cultivate) corrupt or disordered human desire.
[47] Caird, *Principalities and Powers*, 9. See also Berkhof, *Christ and the Powers*, 30.
[48] Berkhof, *Christ and the* Powers, 32.
[49] Yoder, *Politics of Jesus*, 144.
[50] Nicholas Lash, *The Beginning and the End of "Religion,"* 37.
[51] Berkhof, *Christ and the* Powers, 34.
[52] Yoder, *Politics of Jesus*, 147.
[53] Berkhof, *Christ and the Powers*, 38.
[54] Caird, *Principalities and Powers*, 28, is helpful here when he explains that the redemption of the Powers, like the redemption of the Christian, is effected by the cross, and that redemption, or salvation, "is always a past fact, a present experience, and a future hope" (81).
[55] Berkhof, *Christ and the Powers*, 29, italics original.
[56] Yoder, *Politics of Jesus*, 153.
[57] Berkhof, *Christ and the Powers*, 44.
[58] Arthur C. McGill, *Death and Life: An American Theology* (Philadelphia: Fortress, 1987), 18.
[59] Lash, *The Beginning and the End of "Religion,"* 20.
[60] McGill, *Death and Life*, 39.
[61] Self-described Christians are every bit as guilty of this tendency as proud secularists. Vigen Guroian, drawing on the work of Phillipe Aries and Sherwin Nuland, claims: "Even self consciously religious people tend to respond to death with an other-worldliness that suggests a weakened belief in Providence and no real sense of grace. . . . In many cases, the art of caring for the dying has given way to an art of saving life at all cost. (Nuland) adds that this new science of saving life is mostly concerned with the physician's need to be in control and the patient's need to feel that someone is in control." From Vigen Guroian, *Life's Living toward Dying* (Grand Rapids: William B. Eerdmans, 1996), 12-14.
[62] Here see Gerald McKenny, *To Relieve the Human Condition* (Albany: SUNY Press, 1997).
[63] Caird, *Principalities and* Powers, 55.

[64] I am grateful to Steve Bilynskyj for calling attention to the fact that it is suffering, a product of contingency in a fallen creation, and not contingency as such, with which I should be concerned here.
[65] Caird, *Principalities and Powers*, 62.
[66] A somewhat different version of this lecture was presented as the Price Lecture at Wingate University in February 2006. That version will appear in the forthcoming book, *Places of God: Theological Conversations with Wendell Berry*, edited by L. Roger Owens and me.
[67] Ibid., 270.
[68] Ibid., 271.
[69] For a fuller account of Descartes' method and its effect on the way that method leads us to think about the body, see my *The Body of Compassion* (Boulder: Westview, 1999), 15-21.
[70] Alasdair MacIntyre rightly shows that such dualisms as are the heritage of Cartesian philosophy and contemporary reductionist materialism are but part of the same way of regarding the body. See Alasdair MacIntyre, "Medicine Aimed at the Care of Persons Rather Than What . . .?" in *Philosophical Medical Ethics: Its Nature and Significance*, ed. S. F Spicker and H. T. Engelhardt (Doredrecht, Holland: D. Reidel Publishing, 1977), 89.
[71] Here see Drew Lederer, *The Absent Body* (Chicago: University of Chicago Press, 1990). Although he is ultimately not sympathetic with Cartesian dualism, Lederer maintains that on a strictly phenomenological basis the lived experience of "bodily absence," especially common in modern "Western" culture, supports something like the Cartesian position.
[72] Wendell Berry, "Health as Membership," in *Another Turn of the Crank*, 94.
[73] Ibid., 94-95.
[74] Ibid., 96.
[75] Wendell Berry, "Feminism, the Body and the Machine," in *What Are People For?* (New York: North Point, 1990), 190-191; "Discipline and Hope," in *A Continuous Harmony* (New York: Harcourt & Brace, 1972), 147.
[76] Berry, "The Body and the Earth," 280-281.

[77] Berry, "Health as Membership," 90.
[78] Berry, "Healing," in *What Are People For?*, 9.
[79] In the United States, we spend more on medicine than anywhere else in the world. This is the case in absolute terms, per capita, and as a percentage of the gross domestic product.
[80] I am aware that this could well be said of *all* learning, insofar as the acquisition of knowledge is always dependent on the senses. In this case, I am using the expression "using the body" against the background of a kind of rough and ready practical distinction between body and mind that I would not wish to defend as more than heuristic.
[81] Kathleen Norris, *Quotidian Mysteries* (New York: Paulist, 1998).
[82] Here I find useful the point made by Bill Cavanaugh, who follows Michel de Certeau in his distinction between the ways the medieval itinerary and the modern map configure space. Itineraries, he says "told 'spatial stories'," while maps remove the itinerant and rationalize space as homogenous, rendering the particular history irrelevant. "The World in a Wafer: A Geography of the Eucharist as Resistance to Globalization," *Modern Theology* 15:2 (April 1999): 183.
[83] Wendell Berry, "Conservation and Local Economy," in *Sex, Economy, Freedom & Community* (New York: Pantheon, 1993), 3.
[84] Berry, "An Argument for Diversity," in *What Are People For?*, 115.
[85] Leviticus 25:23-24.
[86] Berry, "God and Country," in *What Are People For?*, 99.
[87] Berry, "Christianity and the Survival of Creation," in *Sex, Economy, Community & Freedom*, 98.
[88] Berry, "Word and Flesh" in *What Are People For?*, 200.
[89] On this point, see Karl Barth, *Church Dogmatics*, III/4, trans. A. T. Mackay, et al. (Edinburgh: T & T Clark, 1961), 356-357.
[90] Berry, "Health as Membership," 103.
[91] Barth, *Church Dogmatics*, III/4, 327; 342.
[92] Ibid., 371.
[93] 1 Corinthians 15:54-57.
[94] Berry, "Discipline and Hope," 147.

[95] Berry, "Health as Membership," 105.
[96] Berry, "Damage" in *What Are People For?,* 5.
[97] Ibid.
[98] Ibid.
[99] Berry, "Christianity and the Survival of Creation," 104.
[100] William Cavanaugh, *Theopolitical Imagination* (New York: T & T Clark, 2002), 13.
[101] The classical source for explicating the last part of this claim is Athanasius, *On the Incarnation of the Word of God* (Willits, CA: Eastern Orthodox Books).
[102] Cavanaugh, *Theopolitical Imagination*, 13.
[103] John Zizioulas, *Being as Communion* (Crestwood: SVS Press, 1985), 56.
[104] John Howard Yoder, *Body Politics* (Scottdale: Herald Press, 1992), ix; cf. 28-33.
[105] Eberhard Busch, *Karl Barth: His Life from Letters and Autobiographical Texts*, trans. John Bowden (Philadelphia: Fortress, 1976), 499.
[106] Ernest Becker, *The Denial of Death* (New York: Free Press, 1973).
[107] Ibid., see especially 4-24.
[108] Leo Tolstoy, *The Death of Ivan Ilych and Other Stories* (New York: Signet, 1960), 129.
[109] Ibid.
[110] Emphasis mine.
[111] Ibid., 97.
[112] Ibid., 102.
[113] Becker is, of course, scarcely unique in understanding the terror of death as the essence of the human predicament. On this matter he develops a stream of existentialist and psychoanalytic thought with its origins in the work of thinkers ranging from Kierkegaard to Freud to Adler to Otto Rank.
[114] Becker, *The Denial of Death*, 23.
[115] Wendell Berry, "Manifesto: The Mad Farmer Liberation Front," in *The Selected Poems of Wendell Berry* (Washington: Counterpoint, 1998), 87.

[116] Significantly, Becker follows Kierkegaard in also allowing that a denial of creatureliness (or finitude, if you prefer) can take the form of overt, angry rebellion. See Becker, *The Denial of Death*, 84.
[117] Ibid., 89.
[118] Ibid., 90.
[119] Dante Alighieri, *The Divine Comedy*, trans. John Ciardi (New York: New American Library, 2003). *Inferno*, 1.1-6.
[120] Søren Kierkegaard, *The Concept of Dread* (Princeton: Princeton University Press, 1957), 145. Cited in Becker, *The Denial of Death*, 92.
[121] Robert Pogue Harrison, *The Dominion of the Dead* (Chicago: The University of Chicago Press, 2003), 32.
[122] Ibid.
[123] Ibid., 107.
[124] Romans 6:5.
[125] Harrison, *The Dominion of the Dead*, 110-111.
[126] One could very well expand this list nearly *ad infinitum* by including all of those things that place people at enmity with each other.
[127] Harrison, *The Dominion of the Dead*, 118.
[128] Ibid.
[129] I offer largely the same reading of this story in the book I wrote with Keith Meador, *Heal Thyself: Spirituality, Medicine, and the Distortion of Christianity* (New York: Oxford University Press, 2003), 133-135.
[130] Wendell Berry, "Fidelity," in *Fidelity: Five Stories* (New York: Pantheon, 1992), 107.
[131] Ibid., 113.

THE J.J. THIESSEN LECTURES

A fall lecture series held annually since 1978 at Canadian Mennonite Bible College, Winnipeg, Manitoba, since 2000 at Canadian Mennonite University.

1978 Marlin Miller, Professor of Theology at Goshen (Indiana) Biblical Seminary. *Mennonites and Contemporary Theology.*

1979 *Lectures cancelled.*

1980 J. Gerald Janzen, Professor of Old Testament at Christian Theological Seminary, Indianapolis, Indiana. *The Terrors of History and the Fear of the Lord.*

1981 Frank H. Epp, Professor of History at Conrad Grebel College, Waterloo Ontario. *Mennonites with the Millennium on Their Mind.*

1982 Jürgen Moltmann, Professor of Systematic Theology at the University of Tübingen, Germany. *Responsibility for the World and Christian Discipleship.*

1983 Cornelius J. Dyck, Professor of Anabaptist and Sixteenth Century Studies at Associated Mennonite Biblical Seminaries, Elkhart, Indiana. *Rethinking the Anabaptist Vision.*

1984 Kenneth Bailey, Professor of New Testament at the Near East School of Theology, Beirut, Lebanon. *Jesus Interprets His Own Cross: A Middle Eastern Cultural Approach.*

1985 Orlando Costas, Professor of Missiology at Andover Newton Theological School, Cambridge, Massachusetts. *The Crisis of Mission in the West and the Challenge of World Missions.*

1986 Susan Muto, Director of the Institute of Formative Spirituality at Duquesne University, Pittsburgh, Pennsylvania. *Christian Spirituality and Everyday Living: A Practical Approach to Faith Formation.*

1987 Walter Klaassen, Research Professor of Religious Studies and History at Conrad Grebel College, Waterloo, Ontario. *The Emancipated Laity: Anabaptism in Its Time*

1988 W. Sibley Towner, Professor of Old Testament at Union Theological Seminary, Richmond, Virginia. *The Bible and Our Human Nature.*

1989 Stanley Hauerwas, Professor of Theology and Ethics at the Divinity School, Duke University, Durham, North Carolina. *Resident Aliens: The Church and Its Ministry.*

1990 Werner O. Packull, Professor of History at Conrad Grebel College, Waterloo, Ontario. *Rereading Anabaptist Beginnings.*

1991 I. Howard Marshall, Professor of New Testament at the University of Aberdeen, Scotland. *The Theological Message of the Letter to the Philippians.*

1992 George Lindbeck, Professor at Yale Divinity School, New Haven, Connecticut. *The Church as Hermeneutical Community: Jews, Christians and the Bible.*

1993 Phyllis A. Bird, Associate Professor of Old Testament Interpretation at Garret-Evangelical Theological Seminary, Chicago, Illinois. *Feminism and the Bible.*

1994 David Augsburger, Professor of Pastoral Counselling at Fuller Theological Seminary, Pasadena, California. *Shepherding, Reconciling, Healing: The Church and Christian Counselling.*

1995 George Rawlyk, Professor in the Department of History, Queen's University, Kingston, Ontario. *Is Jesus Your Personal Saviour? In Search of Canadian Evangelicalism in the 1990s.*

1996 Nancey Murphy, Associate Professor of Christian Philosophy at Fuller Theological Seminary, Pasadena, California. *Christian Faith in a Scientific Age.*

1997 Richard B. Hays, Professor of New Testament at Duke Divinity School, Durham, North Carolina. *New Testament Ethics: The Story Retold.*

1998 Eugene H. Peterson, James M. Houston Professor of Spiritual Theology at Regent College, Vancouver, British Columbia. *Christ Plays in Ten Thousand Places.*

1999 T.D. Regehr, Professor Emeritus of History, University of Saskatchewan, Saskatoon, Saskatchewan. *Peace, Order and Good Government: Mennonites and Politics in Canada.*

2000 William P. Brown, Professor of Old Testament at Union Theological Seminary, Richmond, Virginia. *God and the Imagination: A Primer to Reading the Psalms in an Age of Pluralism.*

2001 Letty M. Russell, Professor of Theology, Yale Divinity School, New Haven, Connecticut. *Practicing God's Hospitality in a World of Difference.*

2002 Sean Freyne, Professor of Theology and Director of the Centre for Mediterranean and Near Eastern Studies, Trinity College, Dublin. *Jesus, Jews, and Galilee.*

2003 Paul G. Hiebert, Professor of Mission and Anthropology at Trinity Evangelical Divinity School, Deerfield, Illinois. *Doing Missional Theology.*

2004 Peter C. Erb, Professor of Religion and Culture at Wilfred Laurier University, Waterloo, Ontario. *Late Medieval Spirituality and the Sources for Peace and Reconciliation.*

2005 Paul J. Griffiths, Schmitt Professor of Catholic Studies, University of Illinois at Chicago, Illinois. *The Vice of Curiosity: An Essay on Intellectual Appetite.*

2006 Joel J. Shuman, Associate Professor and Chair of the Department of Theology, and Director of the Center for Ethics and Public Life at King's College in Wilkes-Barre, Pennsylvania. *To Live Is to Worship: Bioethics and the Body of Christ.*